DO IT YOURSELF!

Massage away tension, pain, and many other physical and mental disorders. There is nothing difficult or complicated about the zone therapy techniques described in this book. All but a few professional systems can be performed by anyone.

And zone therapy is perfectly safe. Our techniques may be used alone or in conjunction with conventional medical procedures. Of course, you should always consult your physician in case of serious or persistent symptoms. You may find that zone therapy is just what the doctor ordered.

Just follow our easy instructions. You'll be amazed at the results!

Also by Anika Bergson and Vladimir Tuchak:
SHIATZU

ZONE THERAPY

by Anika Bergson
and Vladimir Tuchak

PINNACLE BOOKS   NEW YORK

ATTENTION: SCHOOLS AND CORPORATIONS

PINNACLE Books are available at quantity discounts with bulk purchases for educational, business or special promotional use. For further details, please write to: SPECIAL SALES MANAGER, Pinnacle Books, Inc., 1430 Broadway, New York NY 10018.

ZONE THERAPY

Copyright © 1974 by Anika Bergson and Vladimir Tuchak

All rights reserved, including the right to reproduce this book or portions thereof in any form.

A Pinnacle Books edition, published for the first time anywhere.

First printing / September 1974

Cover illustration by Bill Maughan

Printed in the United States of America

PINNACLE BOOKS, INC.
1430 Broadway
New York, New York 10018

CONTENTS

	INTRODUCTION	1
1.	HISTORY, ANCIENT AND RECENT	9
2.	OF FEET AND HANDS, OF CHARTS AND TOOLS	19
3.	ANEMIA	27
4.	ANESTHESIA	31
5.	APPENDICITIS	39
6.	ARTHRITIS	43
7.	ASTHMA, BRONCHITIS, COUGHS	47
8.	BACK PROBLEMS, LUMBAGO	53
9.	BLADDER PROBLEMS	59
10.	BLOOD PRESSURE	63
11.	COLDS, SINUSITIS, HAY FEVER	65
12.	DIABETES	69
13.	EAR PROBLEMS, DEAFNESS	71
14.	EPILEPSY	75
15.	EYE PROBLEMS	77
16.	FATIGUE AND DEPRESSION	81
17.	CHILDBIRTH, MORNING SICKNESS, MENOPAUSE, MENSTRUAL CRAMPS	83
18.	GALLBLADDER	91
19.	GOITER	95
20.	HEADACHES, MIGRAINE	97
21.	HEART DISORDERS	99
22.	HEMORRHOIDS	103
23.	HICCOUGHS	105
24.	INFECTIONS, LYMPH GLANDS, KIDNEYS	107
25.	INSOMNIA	109

26.	JOINT PAINS	111
27.	NERVOUSNESS	113
28.	NEURALGIA	117
29.	NEURITIS	119
30.	PARALYSIS, STROKES	121
31.	PNEUMONIA	123
32.	PROSTATE PROBLEMS	125
33.	RECTUM DISORDERS, PROLAPSED RECTUM	129
34.	RELAXATION	131
35.	RHEUMATISM	133
36.	SCIATICA	135
37.	SORE THROAT, LOSS OF VOICE	139
38.	STOMACH DISORDERS	141
39.	TESTES	143
40.	VARICOSE VEINS, LEG CRAMPS	145
41.	PREVENTIVE THERAPY—TEN MINUTES A DAY TO HEALTH	147

ZONE THERAPY

Introduction

This is, to our knowledge, the first book to bring together and collate all the diverse materials involving therapy by means of direct applied pressure on certain key parts of the human body, especially hands and feet. Many books in the past have presented excellent, though partial approaches to this unique science, but no effort has ever been made to synchronize and compare such diverse systems as acupuncture, foot and hand reflexology, and finger and tool massage therapy according to zones. Here then, for the first time, is a book that explains the different approaches, compares them, shows where they agree and where they disagree and, most important, gives the layman and the professional alike a step-by-step guide to the application of a group of systems which have been found to control and alleviate pain and disease in case after case.

The decision to undertake this project was based on the enthusiasm of our own experience with these simple and relatively unknown methods. After years of practicing zone therapy systems daily on a preventive basis, and also in the application of these methods for specific ailments on ourselves, our families, and willing and thankful friends, we felt it was time to pass such information on to the public. Friends who have benefited from our ministrations have been asking us for years to forego the easy life for a time and put down all we know in black and white. In doing so, of course, we have had to borrow from the work and the ideas of the many pioneers in such therapy. We cannot claim that these ideas are original with us; indeed, some of them go back to the ancient Egyptians, and others are the discoveries of the Chinese and the Japanese. The generic term *zone therapy* was coined by Dr. Edwin F. Bowers, M.D., an early associate of the great Dr. William H. FitzGerald, M.D., the first American to attempt to systematize the series of pressure relations he had found in the course of treating his patients and applying anesthesia without opiates in the first decades of this century.

For the sake of objectivity, we have refrained from cluttering the book with personal anecdotes and accounts of miraculous case history cures that do nothing for the reader but impose on his credibility. Instead, we sincerely urge the reader to practice whatever steps we outline as required to benefit his condition, and to practice them consistently and to the letter. If we indicate that four minutes of pressure must be applied on such and such a spot three times a day for so many weeks, we do not mean that two minutes every other day are going to do things for him. And, of course, in this life nothing can be really guaranteed. Even the most conscientious application of these methods might not yield the desired results, especially if the condition is tied to other pathological factors. We might establish a rule of thumb (no pun intended) that if this therapy does not work for a specific and clearly outlined condition, a physician should be consulted immediately, because it is obvious that the situation is such as to require prompt medical attention. We can go further and say that it is good common sense to always undertake the amelioration of any ailment in conjunction with a progressive medical person sympathetic to nonsurgical methods in medicine. Our great hope, naturally, is that in addition to reaching many among the general public suffering from those conditions mentioned in this book, we can bring these techniques to the attention of the medical profession so that, as in the days of Dr. FitzGerald, some real work can again be undertaken by doctors to alleviate even the most serious of conditions through zone therapy systems.

We have sought to bring all pertinent material up to date and to discuss it in an intelligent manner. The avoidance of case history after case history was one way to achieve this. Too often, books on health written on the periphery of the medical profession have tended to sound like the work of quacks, with their fanatical belief in their own narrow and unscientific ways. These books are chatty, repetitive, sometimes confusing, and usually chockfull of unproved statements and facile explanations. The truth is that, to this day, no one knows why this type of therapy works at all. In recent years the West has finally accepted the irrefutable proofs of acupuncture healing in many areas of disease, much to the discomfort of those souls who who can only believe in more "logical" ways. Soviet advances in Kirlian photography have revolutionized the approach to biology and pathology. Such findings, right before the eyes of the world in color photography, support the ancient Chinese concept of Ch'i energy, and take the use of pressure or needles applied on key areas of the body out of the realm of magic. Our work cannot any longer be relegated by anybody to the dustbin of an old wives' tale. Still, the fact remains that zones and meridians have not been explained to the satisfaction of science. The thing works, but no one knows how. Nobody knows for sure why proper pressure below the big toe affects the spinal column at shoulder level. All attempts to say that "crystal deposits" at the nerve endings of the foot are dissolved by pressure, thereby activating blood circulation, are mere conjecture. They are an insult to the scientifically trained person, tending to antagonize him and make him dismiss this whole body of knowledge as pure wishful thinking. We shall offer no pseudoscientific explanations whatever; instead, we shall take a purely pragmatic approach. What works, works, and if it alleviates human suffering, we suggest that it should be practiced whether or not we understand it from the point of view of established science. Someday the actual reasons will be discovered, and we venture to say that they will make as much sense as any other scientific fact. But until then we must limit ourselves to the humble task of showing how to obtain relief from dozens of painful conditions, and that alone.

This is truly a do-it-yourself book. There is nothing complicated or difficult about the techniques in these systems of therapy. Whether you have a professional or just a friend treat you, or you are entirely alone, there are no techniques discussed here that are beyond the grasp and mastery of the layman. A few exceptions are clearly indicated as such and are included in this book for the sake of completeness. For example, throat and nasal massage with the aid of medical tools are mentioned at the appropriate places so that interested doctors may begin to practice again what doctors such as Dr. FitzGerald and Dr. Bowers knew and practiced fifty years ago with great success. Aside from these professional techniques, everything else can be undertaken with complete confidence by the most untrained of persons. We have taken care to go into every detail, the description and portrayal of zones, the comparisons, the precise way to apply pressure, the use of such tools as clothespins, rubber bands, combs, and pencil erasers, and the amount of time required for each operation. There is no way that an error can be made if our instructions are followed. Besides, there is no known danger in practicing these systems even where one fails to do it properly. Body reflexes are such that their manipulation will operate for the benefit of their correlative zones even if we fail to zero in on a malady.

Many charts accompany the text and take the guesswork out of finger and tool massage. With one glance at the appropriate illustration, the neophyte is ready to bring physical relief to himself or those around him. These manipulations are so simple that they can be undertaken standing, sitting, or lying in bed, whichever is the most comfortable.

An important feature of this work is the arrangement and discussion according to areas and ailments to be treated. Most books on the subject treat these things in a less direct fashion, preferring to discuss several things at once or suddenly coming forth with gratuitous advice on other matters, with the result that the reader has to wade through reams of material before coming upon and understanding that which most interests him. In this book, beginning with Chapter Three, zone therapy systems are broken down alphabetically by disease or area of discomfort. This allows quick reference. If you suffer from headaches you can open the book to the chapter on headaches;

you won't find anything there about the gallbladder to confuse you and delay the treatment.

Naturally, a book devoted to the study of so mysterious and together a thing as the human body could not end on a divisive note. When a part or an organ of the body has been suffering from a pathological condition, it doesn't take long before affecting other parts and organs. An ounce of prevention is therefore worth a pound of regret. Consequently, the reader's attention is directed to the last chapter, Ten Minutes to Health. There he will find a discussion of preventive medicine and of the simple therapy he can follow to retain and improve his health. It is ironic that millions of people practice muscle exercises religiously each morning upon arising, as if their bodies were entirely made up of muscle and nothing but muscle. Now, we are not for one minute suggesting that such an excellent practice be discontinued. On the contrary, muscle tone is one of the keys to general body health. Unfortunately for these people, it is far from being the whole story. Such exercises should be backed up by the equally important exercise of glands and internal organs. Only zone therapy systems can reach these all-important centers of life. It is entirely up to the individual just how healthy he wishes to be once he is acquainted with the secrets of radiant well-being. The exercise we have devised for either morning or evening application take no longer than ten minutes to perform. It may yield dividends measurable in years of happy life and contented old age.

It is primarily as a preventive and additional therapy that this book is offered to the general public. No claim is made by the authors that any technique described here will work in any specific case. Indeed, not even medical science can claim to cure each and every case that comes to its attention. Zone therapy systems are meant to be applied side by side with the thoughtful ministrations of your own physician; they should have his supervision and meet with his approval. Zone therapy systems are a boost to conventional curative methods as practiced by the medical profession, not something opposed to or at variance with its practice. What can be said to be true is that the conscientious application of the techniques described in this book can bring relief of harmful tensions and other dangerous psychosomatic factors. Where this, plus the relief of pain, is achieved, we are well on the road to recovery and the defeat of disease.

The stark simplicity of these wonderful methods stands in direct and dramatic contrast to the very nature of disease and those stubborn and depressing psychological conditions which disease brings in its wake. Zone therapy systems cannot possibly be detrimental if followed correctly. They can be amazingly, miraculously effective.

1

History, Ancient and Recent

There is almost no doubt that some very ancient civilizations knew how to cure the diseases of man in ways that would certainly amaze us, and make us grope for adjectives other than crude or primitive. Chance and experimentation with massage, pressure, herbs, and diet throughout thousands of years must have led in a good many cases to great finds, to discoveries that helped prove a boon to mankind. Then, of course, these civilizations decayed or were overrun, and their medical secrets were lost or destroyed. Perhaps some survive to this day, and each one of us has scoffed at what we deprecatingly call old wives' tales, handed down by word of mouth since time immemorial, not sure that they work and unwilling to try them. Willful cases involving the destruction of knowledge, such as the tragic burning of the library at Alexandria or the destruction of a wonderful body of Indian herbal lore by the Spaniards, are incalculable historical losses. Events of this nature can be blamed for the little we know, for instance, of how the ancient

Egyptians practiced medicine, or how the Incas managed brain surgery. In those cases where we are believed to have better records, such as with Chinese folk medicine, we discover that the curtain of fog parts to reveal not so much facts as myths about its origins. This cannot be avoided, for ancient man saw all events impinging on his destiny within the context of magic and religion. The concepts of traditional Chinese medicine and acupuncture are intimately connected with the philosophy of the *Tao Te Ching*, or Book of the Way. Especially important concepts are those of yin and yang, and the notion that man—as indeed all things—exists in a vast and indivisible whole which is constantly interreacting. The ancient Chinese sages believed that for man to maintain mental and physical health he had to enter into a harmonious relationship with everything else; he had to fit into a world of correspondences where the twin principles, yin and yang, ruled "the ten thousand things." Yin represents the negative force, the quiescent, female principle; and yang the positive, active, male principle. Just how these two principles are balanced in one's body would explain to the Chinese sage one's state of health. For instance, where yang is predominant, the body tends to be overheated, fevers have a chance to rise, the person is tense and irritable.

It should be obvious that with such an all-encompassing approach, even the most ancient Chinese doctors could do much for their patients; certainly much more than their European counterparts of the Middle Ages. Chinese history is replete with the names of great doctors and their cures. Magnificent finds, such as the circulation of the blood, are mentioned in the *Huang-ti nei ching*, or The Yellow Emperor's Book of Internal Medicine, some 4,000 years ago.

Acupuncture, conservatively estimated to be more than 2,000 years old, is based on the concept that the human body has an internal set of channels—or meridians, as these are now called—with 365 points where the channels surface onto the skin. These meridians are places where control on yin and yang can best be exercised and effected by the insertion of needles.

Up to the turn of this century, acupuncture was practiced exclusively in the Orient; yet, curiously enough, Western doctors in the nineteenth century had begun to discover hitherto hidden secrets about the human body that were not too unlike what the Chinese knew empirically. The earliest to do so was the Swede Pehr Henrik Ling. In 1834, Ling noticed that pains emanating from certain organs were reflected in certain areas of the skin with no direct relation to those organs. Other students followed, including the English neurologist Sir Henry Head; the treatment zones he discovered came to be known as "Head's zones." Therapeutic anesthesia had been born. Today, we are beginning to find how these zones bear relationships to acupuncture, even though the complexity of the nervous system is one that will continue to baffle scientists looking for clear-cut "reasons" for all this seeming nonsense. But research scientists are in agreement that, when all is said and done, yin and yang polarities correspond to our Western theory of the sympathetic and parasympathetic nervous system.

The recent work done in the Soviet Union, especially by S. D. Kirlian and V. Kh. Kirlian, is of outstanding importance because it tends to prove the reality of meridians and, by implication, the entire theory of zone therapy systems. As far back as the 1890s, a Russian engineer named Yakov Narkevich-Todko was experimenting with electrographic photographs. These were obtained by using electrical discharges to photograph weird bluish flames emanating from living bodies. These bluish discharges have been known since Biblical times, and are most familiar to sailors because they are often seen around the mastheads and the riggings of ships. This phenomenon is commonly called St. Elmo's fire. It occurs on land as well, and records exist of people out West reporting opening their iron stoves only to see a big bluish ball of fire come tumbling out. There is a simple explanation for this: the stove chimney probably attracted static electricity, available whenever there are electrical storms in the air. The electricity, accumulating in the bowels of the stove, came out as a ball of flame.

Stranger still, cases have been reported where human beings have seemed to act as storage batteries for this kind of electricity. Anyone touching them would receive a painful shock.

In any event, as Czechoslovakian parapsychologists suggest, a kind of biological energy, which they have termed bio-energy, is at work in a great deal of so-called psychic phenomena. This bio-energy is far more subtle than electromagnetic waves, and the way it operates within the human body is not yet known. It is there, of that we may be sure, but its relationship to the health of the person is still a puzzle to investigators. What we can assert is that this energy demands that our previous, simplistic, mechanical approach to bodily functions and interactions be expanded, as was Newtonian physics.

Experiments by the Kirlians demonstrate that photographs of the fingertips of an even-tempered man, as opposed to those of a tired, emotionally tense individual, differed not once but consistently as far as those mysterious flames are concerned; and such photographs have been published, showing graphically these remarkable differences. The fact inescapably emerges that living organisms are electrodynamic systems of great complexity, and the most subtle correlations exist between their parts.

As the Kirlians found out when they used their technique to photograph leaves, a healthy leaf will give a different image than an old or a dried-out one. Thus, the biological condition of an organism can be read in the same way that X-rays enable us to read skeletal conditions. From the point of view of preventive medicine, such "readings" will help diagnose conditions which could not otherwise be detected, or discovered as soon. One of the most interesting things that the Kirlians found out was that different parts of the human skin give off different colors. They state that the heart region gives off an intense blue, the forearm is greenish-blue, and the thigh olive green. During fear or illness the inherent color of an area changes. The flames that emanate from the skin are reported to differ; they are not uniform or even. Some come in the shape of points, others form coronas and flares of luminescent clusters that come in different colors. At some points on the skin blue and gold luminescences flare up suddenly. Could these be acupuncture points? Some of these flames leap from one point on the skin only to land on another, where they are absorbed. Scientists assume that these different performance patterns obey different biomechanical systems functioning in common, just as the different colors observed could emanate from different systems.

So complete is the biological entity from the point of view of these electrical systems that when a leaf with a section missing has been photographed, the flare patterns of the entire leaf continue to appear as if that part had not been removed at all and were still part and parcel of the leaf.

Perhaps enough has been said to convince the reader that the next few decades will bring revolutionary changes in the way we go about mending and helping the body back to health. New medical techniques will be used that are not even in their infancy at this point. But the importance of pressure therapy cannot be underestimated in this connection, and we should see a great development in the spread and sophistication with which zone massage is used in pathology as well as in preventive medicine.

Exciting as the prospect appears, we are still back at the stage of creeping doubts and official contention. The American doctors who pioneered zone therapy systems in the early part of this century had to wage an uphill fight not to be laughed out of town as simple charlatans. Even today, the notion of a doctor suggesting that you clench a plain aluminum comb in your hand for some minutes in order to relax you and relieve you of a case of lumbago is so preposterous-sounding that your first impulse is to laugh and go see the medical man next door. And yet, that is precisely what Dr. William FitzGerald was able to do on occasion, with brilliant results.

Dr. FitzGerald was an ear, nose, and throat specialist in Connecticut. He was a graduate of the University of Vermont, who worked in hospitals in Boston, London, and Vienna. He began to be interested in this new approach by observing that he could carry out minor operations on the nose and throat by replacing the cocaine used in those days to deaden pain with pressure on certain parts of the body. Looking into the matter further, he discovered that not all patients reacted alike to these pressures, and that some patients came to him and, either before or during the operation, would tense up or squeeze their hands in preparation for the ordeal they were expecting. In some cases, the tension along the hands was enough to anesthetize these persons. Soon, he had his dentist friends using his method of pressure application in order to perform their previously horrifyingly painful work. Hundreds and hundreds of patients were treated by these men at the dawn of zone therapy systems, some of them with truly amazing results. But, of course, even in the medical profession prejudice dies hard, and doctors by and large preferred to continue believing in their time-honored methods rather than experiment and find drugless solutions to human suffering

One man who was not afraid to look into the matter was Dr. Edwin F. Bowers, M.D., of New York, who took it upon himself to go and visit Dr. FitzGerald and observe for himself some of these cures that were the talk of professional circles. Dr. Bowers left convinced that there was something very important in those methods, and wrote an article in which he christened the budding science zone therapy.

Dr. FitzGerald evolved a theory that divided the human body longitudinally into five zones on the left and five zones on the right. We will be comparing these zones with the meridians of acupuncture in the next chapter, so it will suffice to mention here that these zones relate all parts of the body within each zone in such a way that any problem in one zone could conceivably be treated by pressure somewhere else within it. In this way, a problem with the left eye could react to pressure on the third toe of the left foot, since both these parts of the body lie within zone three. This is, naturally, an oversimplification, because relief will depend upon how and where exactly that toe is pressured, but the explanation has been given for the sake of presenting in capsule form the single most important element in zone therapy systems.

In view of all we have said relating to acupuncture and Kirlian photography, the reader will immediately understand the profound rightness of the theory which Dr. FitzGerald came upon, thanks to his sensitivity to human pain, a sensitivity that marked him as a true physician. Most methods of pressure therapy in the United States stem from the work of those two American pioneers, Dr. FitzGerald and Dr. Bowers, in addition to the incredibly successful practice of the Los Angeles doctor, George Starr White, M.D.

But enough of history. Let's get on with the

task of discovering a few secrets of the human body, and how we can put those secrets to work for us in relieving pain and assisting the curative powers of nature.

2

Of Feet and Hands, of Charts and Tools

A comparison of the chart designed by Dr. FitzGerald (see Figure 1) showing the body divided into five zones on the left and five on the right, with Master H'su Ch'ang's acupuncture meridians (Figure 2) will show how closely related the two approaches are to a general way of treating the human body and its ailments.

Acupuncture has developed a method of treating points where the meridians surface on the body by means of needles inserted at those points. Until recently, there was no scientific proof that these points were any different from any other area in the body, but Dr. Kim Bongham of North Korea has discovered "little groups of egg-shaped cells at acupuncture points which are united with one another by bundles of hollow tubular cells..." So there appears to be this "fourth system of communication—the others being nervous, vascular, and lymphatic."

Only further research will show just how zone therapy as applied to the feet and hands

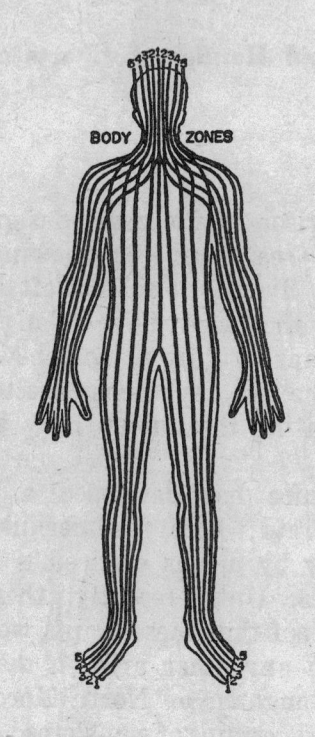

Figure 1.

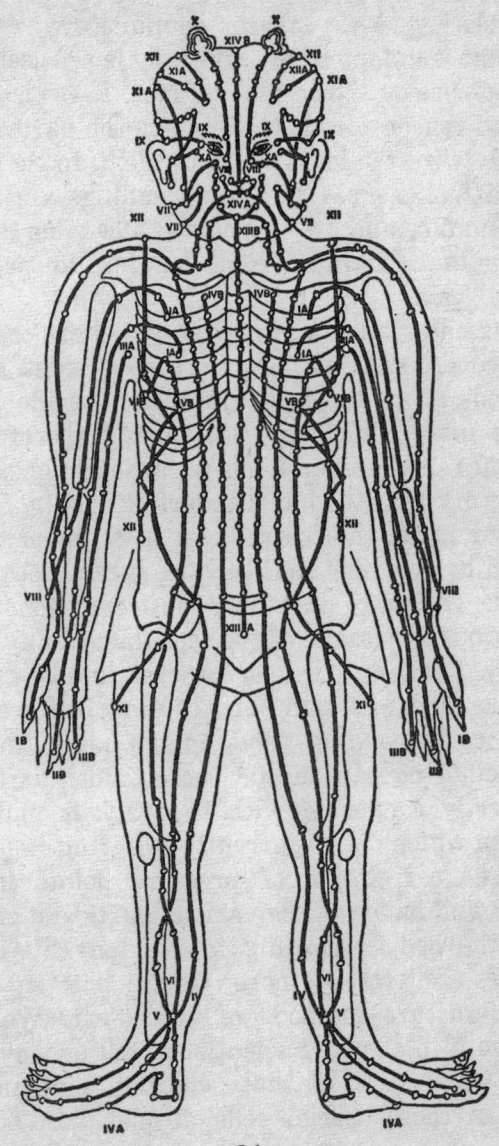

Figure 2.

works vis-à-vis these acupuncture centers. What is unique to zone therapy is precisely that emphasis on the hands and feet. There is a very good reason for this; these are the parts of the body with the least depth to them. In the hands and feet, nerves and nerve endings are forced to surface and are thus more accessible to massage and manipulation, leading to pressure analgesia.

If one studies the FitzGerald chart one soon discovers that the same reflexes exist in the hands as in the feet. However, specific points are more difficult to locate and therefore to treat in the human hand, because of the amount of work that the hand undertakes daily. On the other hand, the foot is kept in a tender condition by the very fact that we wear shoes. It is thus easier to treat the entire system by a thorough massage of the feet than in any other way. Readers will soon discover just how much more tender certain parts of their feet are than the corresponding parts on the hand. And the fascinating part is that those tender parts are directly connected with the various maladies from which one is currently suffering.

The correlation of pressure points in the feet and hands to the various parts and organs of the body according to the ten FitzGerald zones follows a more direct pattern than acupuncture methods of treatment. We will leave it to a future scientist to tell us why that is. Our guess is that whereas acupuncture treats those special cells at meridian points, zone therapy works more directly on nerve endings that are intimately connected with organs along the ten zones.

Leaving aside the more theoretical aspects, we would like at this point to discuss the various simple tools that may be used to relieve pain. Before doing so, however, the reader should study Figures 3 and 4, for these charts give him a bird's-eye view of the zone areas in both the hands and the feet. We will be going into the ways to attack these pressure areas depending on the malady involved, but we suggest that the reader take the first practical step at this time and, chart in hand, follow or feel the various points indicated on both the hands and the feet. Pressure may be applied with the thumb. We venture to say that the average reader will be surprised to find how many areas respond with soreness when only a minimal amount of firm pressure is applied. That is one indication that the reader's health is not as abundant as it should be.

From time to time we will be suggesting a variety of simple tools that may be used in zone therapy. In addition to the all-important human thumb, which is generally the best tool, there will be times when a more incisive pressure will be required. The rubber eraser on a pencil is marvelous for just that kind of fine, in-depth massage required at times. The pioneers in zone therapy discovered early in the game that a more constant kind of pressure on the fingers of the hand worked wonders with

Figure 3.

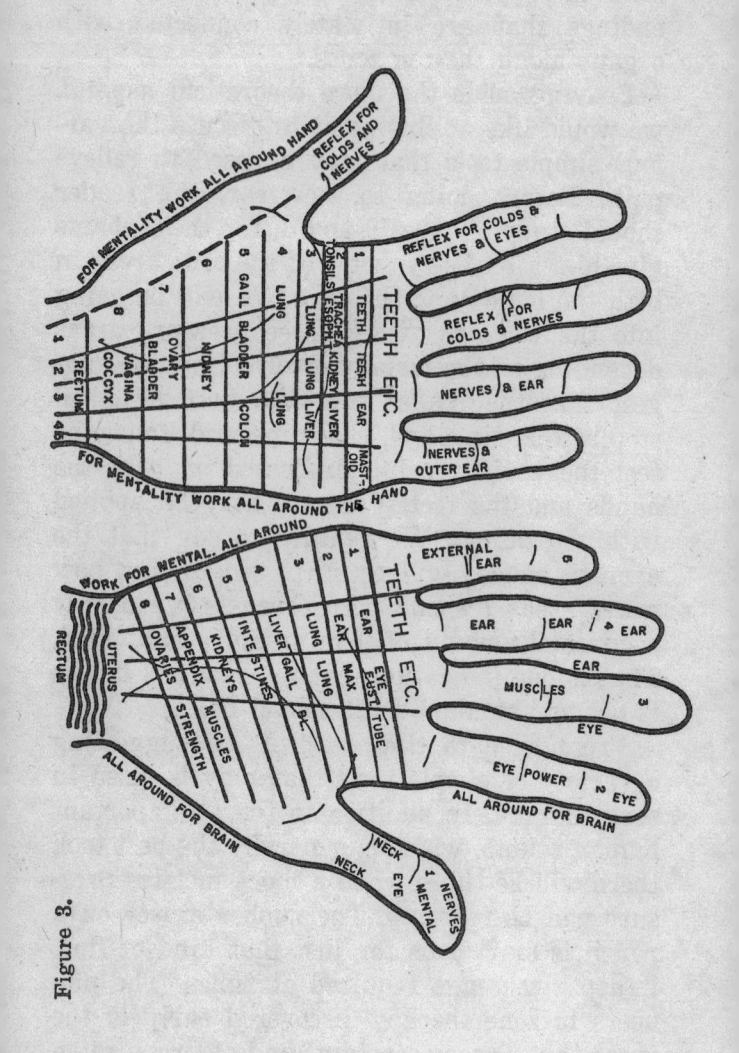

Figure 4.

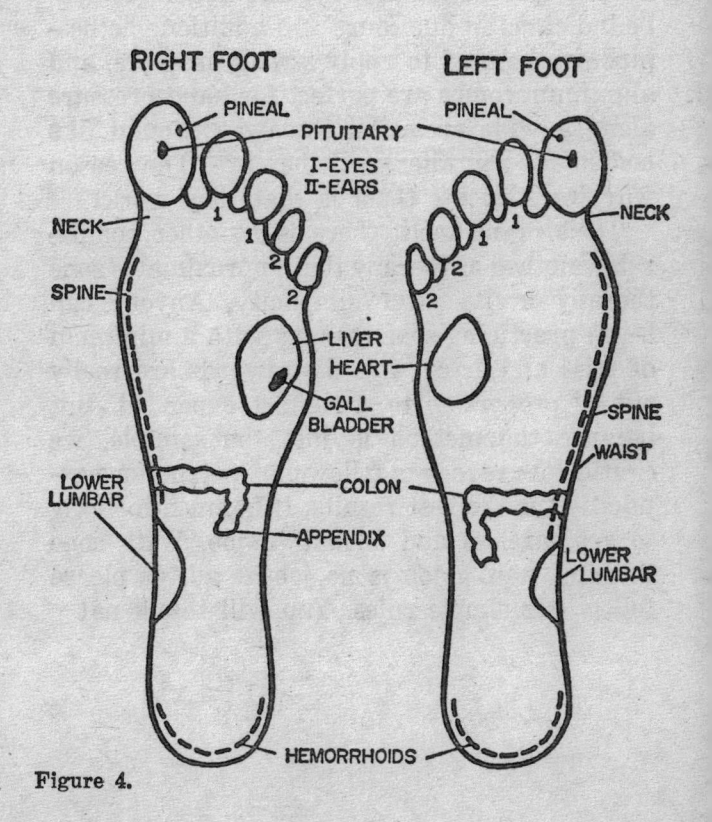

some ailments. Pragmatists that they were, they soon found a perfect solution for that in the form of rubber bands. These are wound around specific joints of specific fingers, as will be indicated in due course. In addition, clothespins can be used to apply strong pressure, and aluminum combs are perfect for hand pressure along a wide area. All these may sound like homemade remedies, and they are. The reason why we advocate them is that they work!

Tools or no tools, there is no other comparable method of therapy that approximates zone therapy in its utter simplicity. Anyone can begin practicing zone therapy with a minimum of trial and error, and the rewards are really out of proportion to the effort expended. But because the method is just that simple, we caution the reader to follow our instructions explicitly for the best results. It is much too easy to get careless and do half a job. With zone therapy, half a job is no job at all, so please follow our simple rules. You will thank us!

3

Anemia

Anemia is due to lack of iron in the blood; it can cause serious trouble if left to run its course. Women, who need more iron than men, are more prone to anemia.

The organ most directly involved with anemia is the spleen, because it is there that iron is stored until needed by the blood. If you discover that the area of the spleen in your foot has any tenderness, you are probably somewhat anemic. Fortunately, improvement can be rapid unless you have pernicious anemia, in which case the cure will be slower.

If you refer to Figure 5, you will see that the spleen lies under the heart, on the left side of the body. Consequently, only the left foot, at the appropriate place, should be massaged.

The spleen is a soft but brittle organ somewhat long and flattened, whose size and weight is liable to vary at different periods in life. The adult spleen is usually about five inches in length and weighs about seven ounces.

Because the spleen has a lot to do with both the large and small intestines, soreness at the

Figure 5.

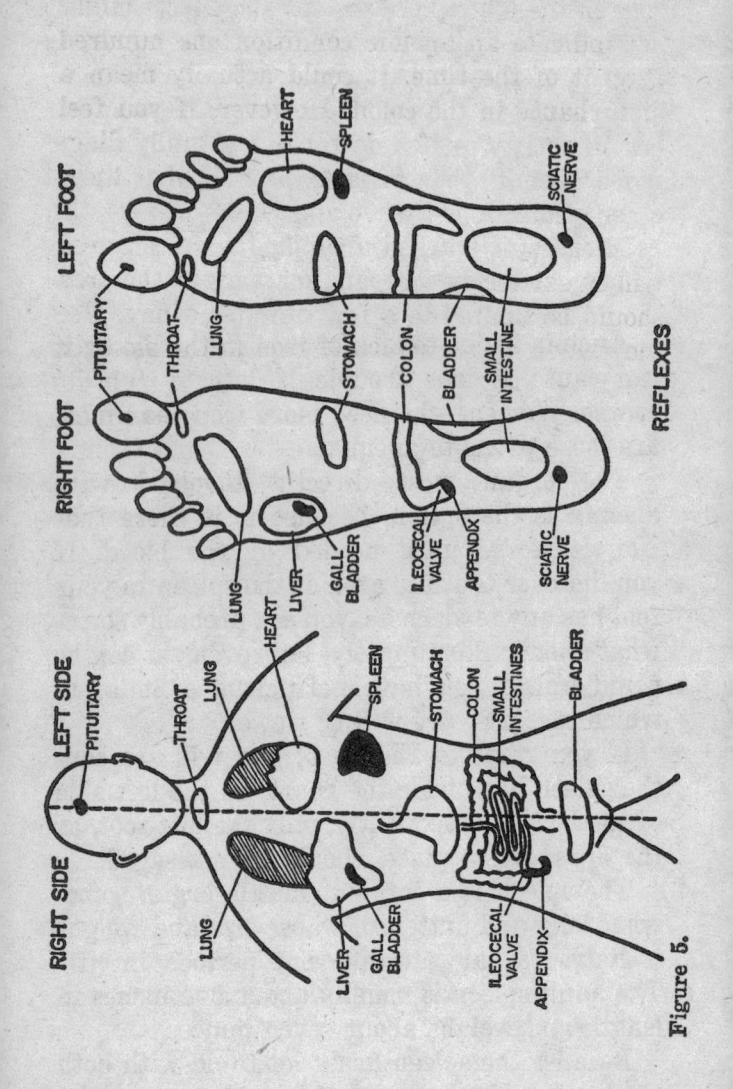

zone in the foot where the spleen reflects might not indicate an anemic condition one hundred percent of the time. It could actually mean a disturbance in the colon. However, if you feel low in energy or if a doctor has actually diagnosed anemia, then you can assume that those other connections do not apply.

In cases of marked anemia, the spleen area will be extremely sore, and massage of the area should be limited to a few minutes a day. Use the thumb in a circular motion directly over the sore spot.

In addition to massage, a diet rich in minerals, as directed by a competent nutritionist, will assist in recovery.

4

Anesthesia

This chapter will be of more interest to doctors and dentists than to the layman, but the subject is of enough importance to warrant appearing in a do-it-yourself type of book such as this.

We should begin by pointing out that there is a difference between zone therapy and what can be termed direct nerve blocking or pressure analgesia. This latter consists—as the term implies—of pressure directly over the nerve supplying a certain area. Obviously, this is quite different from a system that applies pressure in a zone far removed from the area that one is treating.

That both approaches work can be proven by experimentation. Pressure directly on the dental nerve will block sensations normally felt on the teeth involved with that nerve. With zone therapy, pressure on certain fingers or toes in the same zone will inhibit the pain in that same tooth or teeth.

If the reader will refer back to Figure 1, he will see, for instance, that both the big toe and the thumb are in zone one, and that zone one is the most central of the zones and involves the nose, front teeth, center of the tongue, and so on down the body. Similarly, the various toes and fingers affect corresponding parts of the body. Common sense will show that the middle ear, for instance, is in zone four. An organ like the liver lies in all five zones on the right side of the body, and in zones one, two, and sometimes three on the left side; a good practitioner of zone therapy makes sure that he covers all possible zones for a given organ when massaging. Another point we might make at this time is that in treating any of the internal organs it is a good idea to tackle both the anterior and posterior zone simultaneously (see Figures 6 and 7).

Empirical knowledge of anesthesia has existed for a long time. Everyone knows that a blow to the pit of the stomach will render a person unconscious. Fighters are aware that a blow to the temple or at a certain angle to the jaw will produce similar results. In the old days, before anesthesia, surgeons sometimes experimented with pressure along the nerve centers in the neck. The results obtained were positive; however, no one knew how long the patient would remain unconscious after the operation!

Pain anywhere in the first zone can be treated and made to disappear, sometimes for good, through pressure on the entire surface of the big toe's first joint. If the pressure is ap-

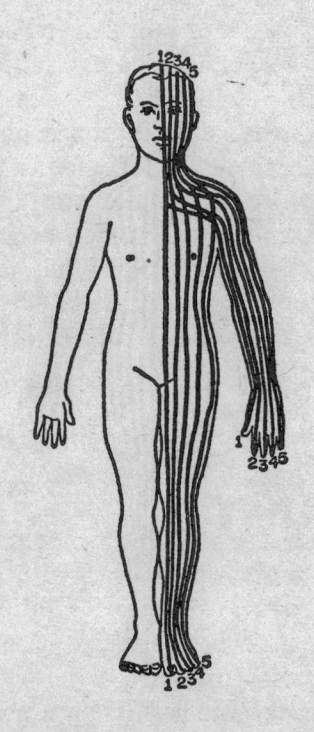

Figure 6.

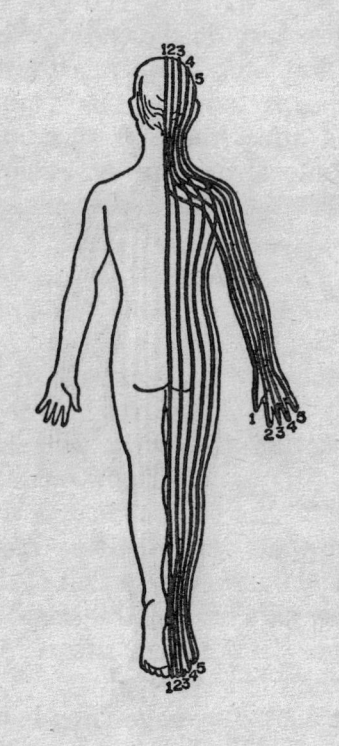

Figure 7.

plied only on the upper surface, the effect will be felt along the front of the body. Conversely, pressure on the under side of the big toe will bring relief along the first zone in back of the body.

Strong pressure on the end of the big toe or the tip of the thumb controls the whole first zone. Similar pressure on the tips of the other fingers will affect the corresponding zones in the body. Lateral pressure on either fingers or toes will affect the lateral boundaries of the body.

Partial anesthesia can also be obtained by pressure on a bony surface. This pressure may be applied with a sharp-pointed applicator or with the nails of the thumb or fingers.

Pressure applied through rubber bands wound on fingers, toes, wrist, or ankle will also produce anesthesia. Even the knees and elbows can be involved in this method so that pain in several zones can be eliminated. One point that we must make, however, is that if the pain increases after this kind of treatment, pathological symptoms of another nature may be involved in the zones affected.

Pressure should average from half a minute to four minutes or longer, depending on the severity of the pain.

Dentists should know that pressure on the big toe may anesthetize the incisor region enough for the painless extraction of incisors and bicuspids. The dentist may supplement this pressure himself by applying pressure directly on the lip or cheek and on the jaw. The second zone usually includes the cuspids and biscuspids. The third zone governs the two molars and the fourth zone the third molar teeth. Pressure applied with the thumb or a cautery contact on the upper or lower jaw will relieve pain by zone.

Dr. FitzGerald gives further advice to dentists as follows: "Pressure or cautery contact on the buccal surface of the jaws control anterior sections of zones, one, two, three, four, and often five; and pressure or cautery contact on lingual surface of jaws control posterior sections of above zones. Zones four and five usually merge in the head. Pressure with the thumb or finger on inferior dental and lingual nerves, at inferior dental foramen, will often anesthetize that half of the jaw, and to a greater extent the entire half of the body on side compressed.

"Because of the anastomosis of nerves at the median line of the jaw, this pressure occasionally causes an anesthesia of a part or even the whole of the opposite side of the jaw, but this is the only instance thus far noticed where anesthesia through pressure crosses the median line of the body."

A mouth in which there is normal occlusion by the natural teeth is a great asset, since the entire organism can be made to relax by simple biting pressure held for two or three minutes. Pain in any zone can sometimes be relieved by this simple expedient; occasionally, even anesthesia may be induced where true occlusion occurs and the pressure is held firmly for a few minutes.

These methods will never produce soreness of the jaw. Quite the contrary, in cases where operations have been carried out or where hemorrhage has taken place, pressure with the thumb or fingers will overcome or lessen the difficulty.

In conclusion, we might sum up this entire question of anesthesia by saying that a practiced doctor or dentist can anesthetize a patient from the head to the feet by pressure on resistant surfaces of the head and/or by pressure on the extremities. Individuals may obtain analgesic effects by means of pressure with their teeth if they possess good occlusion, and by pressure on specific fingers.

It should be pointed out that whereas the right amount of pressure is of great value to the organism, too much pressure, or for too long a period, is harmful and leads to weakness and irritability. Tight shoes, belts, corsets, or collars will invariably have a detrimental effect upon bodily health.

5

Appendicitis

The reflex for the appendix and the ileocecal valve, which connects the small intestine to the large, is located slightly to the right of center on the right foot (see Figure 8). The appendix is a narrow tube from three to six inches long; it has no fixed position. Pressure with the left thumb on the spot indicated can soon tell you

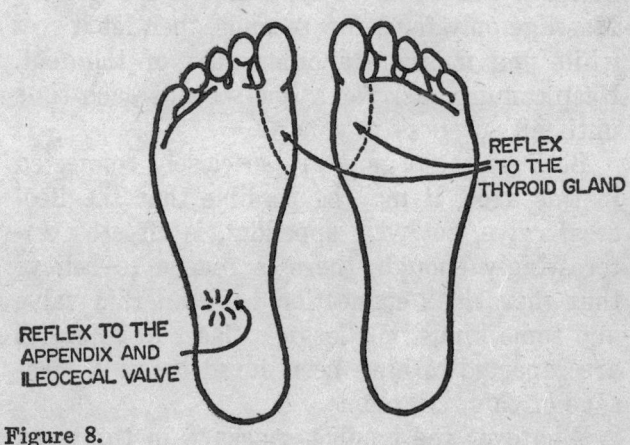

Figure 8.

if there is a tendency to congestion of the appendix.

Recoveries from appendicitis have been achieved through the massaging of the reflex for this organ. However, in case of an acute attack, a physician should be seen at once. You may massage the appendix reflex until he sees you since this action can only benefit the situation, but bear in mind that it won't be a solution.

Since the appendix is a small organ, a little exploring with the thumb will be necessary before you can zero in on it. Press in with the tip of the thumb below the foot's center and slightly toward its outer edge. Now move the thumb in a rolling motion. If you detect some pain there, it might be worthwhile to switch to a pencil with a rubber eraser and explore the exact location of the pain so that the massage will center on the source of the trouble. Massage only for a few seconds, then let it rest while you massage another part of the foot. Keep coming back for a few seconds each time until all soreness is gone.

Because the organs are so closely connected in this area, it may be possible that the ileocecal valve, not your appendix, is affected. Interestingly enough, there is reason to believe that there is a connection between this valve and some kinds of allergies. Cases of allergies are reported to have been cured through massage of this reflex zone.

Whatever the trouble, massage in this area will help relieve symptoms that might be accumulating and which would cause serious trouble later on. The abolition of soreness in this area through careful massage represents a wonderful case of preventive medicine.

6

Arthritis

Arthritis is so complex a condition that not even medical science is able to cope with it. There are many theories about it but nothing is known for certain. Because of this fact, we can only suggest a couple of methods that might bring amelioration.

The first is based on the idea that arthritis is caused by an accumulation of poisons and acids, as well as calcium, and that this is due to faulty functioning of the digestive system. It would do no harm for the person suffering from arthritis to concentrate then on massaging that area of the feet directly connected to the stomach and intestines (see Figure 4), remembering that one cannot expect results with arthritis in days or weeks. Experimentation with the massage in the feet reflexes of the several internal organs might yield an unexpected result. This result might be preceded by an apparent worsening of the arthritic condition as the poisons retained by the system are released through the massage.

The other approach is to attack those reflexes

in the feet connected to the endocrine glands. After all, these are the glands that supply the body with the regulatory factors and substances that bring health. A condition such as arthritis may signify that one gland or another is not delivering or functioning properly. Please study Figure 9 and see that you massage the reflexes to all of them for at least two weeks. The thumb is the best instrument for this and several minutes a day will suffice. When you find a particularly tender spot give it a good massage and come back to it later on. Do one foot at a time and be sure to massage any tender area regardless of its connection to a specific organ. Pain in the foot is always an indication of disorder in the body, so no soreness should be disregarded.

When massaging the parathyroid reflexes, you might wish to transfer to the use of a rubber eraser at the tip of a pencil, since it is necessary to really hit those small spots in the feet, and the thumb is too broad in this case.

Figure 9.

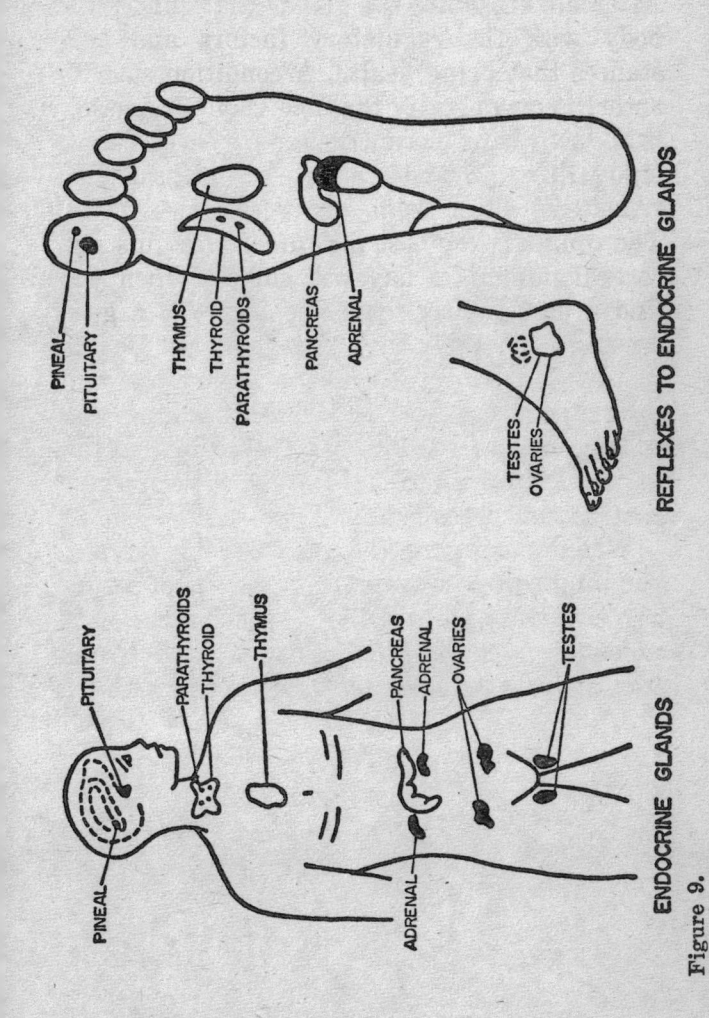

7

Asthma, Bronchitis, Coughs

Asthmatic conditions are best treated by means of pressure on the floor of the mouth. In fact, the old pioneers of zone therapy had many nearly miraculous cures to report by using this direct method of attack. For this purpose, a medical probe that is cotton-tipped works best, and it should be used beneath the root of the tongue.

Severe bronchial asthma may also be relieved by pressing strongly on the first and third zones of the tongue (the tongue contains all ten zones) with a tongue depressor. In fact, patients may help themselves by biting the tongue as hard as possible, holding it between the teeth for several minutes at a time, three or four times daily.

Persons suffering from asthma would do well to have their teeth, throat, and pharynx checked by a medical doctor, since it is a fact that some asthmatic conditions are not resolved until defects in these areas are cleared up.

Some authorities in the field insist that asthma can be treated through zone therapy by attacking the reflex for the adrenal glands (see Figure 9). They base their theory on the fact that since adrenalin injections can help break up an attack of asthma, it should follow that activation of the adrenal glands might just be the thing that will bring on relief of this condition. Asthmatic patients with soreness showing at the point of this reflex will do well to massage it several times a day.

Dr. FitzGerald had several suggestions, some of which can only be undertaken by a physician. In the first place, he suggested traction of the soft palate with a finger or a hook probe. In some cases he found that the use of rubber bands wound around all the fingers or toes, from ten to fifteen minutes several times daily, brought improvement. One of his strangest methods was to press with the index finger against the front teeth of the patient.

For bronchitis, a doctor may pass a cotton-tipped probe through the nose to the epipharynx. When he has touched the exact location, the patient should feel a sensation in his throat that corresponds to the zones of the bronchi affected. Such pressure should be maintained from one to three minutes.

A less extreme method involves the use of the two index fingers to stretch the lips. This should be done several times daily. Coughs may be alleviated by this simple process.

The central zones affected by asthma or cough can also be treated by tongue-pulling (see

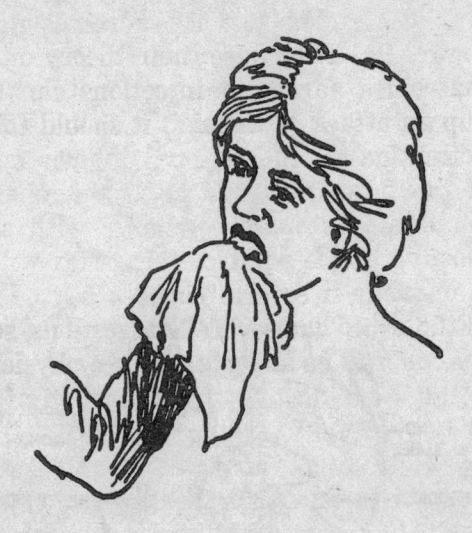

Figure 10.

Figure 10). The tongue may be twisted from side to side as well.

Zone therapy is most directly involved in bronchial cases by the manipulation of the foot reflexes for the lungs and bronchial tubes. These reflexes are located at the pads of the feet, directly beneath the toes (see Figure 11). Since the lungs take up quite a bit of space in the chest, it is not unusual to find that their reflexes in each foot take up so much room. To massage, hold the right foot with the left hand and use the right hand to rub the entire reflex area. Use a circular, rolling motion. Massage of the whole lung area will benefit the bronchial tubes. And since the bronchial tubes are buried deep in the chest, it may be necessary for you to massage

Figure 11.

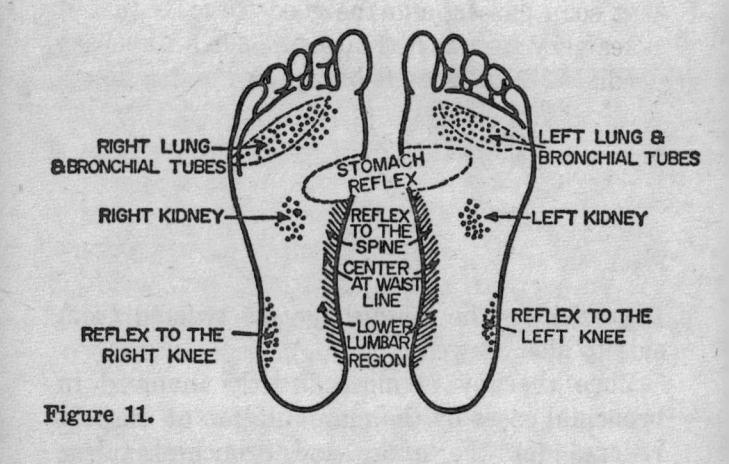

thoroughly and deeply; a light probe may not even reveal soreness.

Whooping coughs and other types of cough may be handled as follows: A cotton-tipped probe is applied to the back of the throat (the post-pharyngeal wall) and held firmly there for several minutes. The throat may develop some soreness from this type of treatment but that soon passes, and the good thing is that it takes very few such treatments for an average condition to clear up. This applies to any cough originating in the respiratory passages in that zone (and not, of course, to something like a tubercular cough).

A less complicated method of curing a cough is to grasp the tongue resolutely (see Figure 10) and give it a long and hard pull, holding it out as long as the patient can stand it.

The use of the probe might scare some people, although we recommend it as the quickest cure of all. Less dramatic results can also be obtained by the application of firm pressure on the front part of the tongue and on the floor of the mouth under the tongue. In addition, moderately tight rubber bands may be worn on the thumbs and first fingers of the hands for five and even ten minutes at a time, several times a day.

Holding the bridge of the nose with the first finger and thumb and applying strong pressure for several minutes is also helpful, especially if there is a frontal headache accompanying the cough.

8

Back Problems, Lumbago

Practically everybody complains at one time or another of pains in the back. Back problems are almost endemic to man and are attributed to the fact that, back in the forgotten past, he changed his way of walking and straightened up, placing a great amount of stress on the small of the back. Be that as it may, zone therapy can help immensely to restore health to any part of the back faced with problems of pinched nerves and the congestion brought on by muscular contraction.

Since the spinal column is in the exact center of the body, it follows that the reflex for it lies along the first zone of each foot (see Figure 12), going lengthwise from the big toe to the heel. If you understand that the toe itself stands for the head and that the center of the foot stands for the center of the back, and so forth, you will have no trouble in locating the exact spot to manipulate in reference to the pains along your back. People with problems in the lumbar region of the spine will follow the reflex down towards the heel until they can lo-

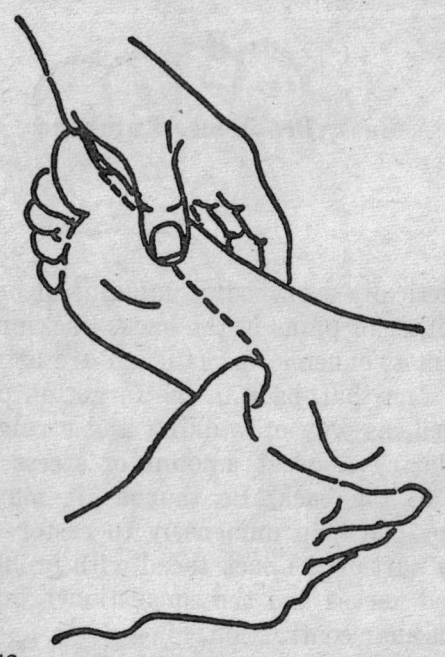

Figure 12.

cate tell-tale tenderness. When the problem area is located, begin your massage quite gently at first—spine reflexes are usually quite sore—and continue in this fashion until you can work the tenderness out.

The reflexes of the back may be massaged for any length of time you desire, unlike certain organs such as the liver, which must be handled with care.

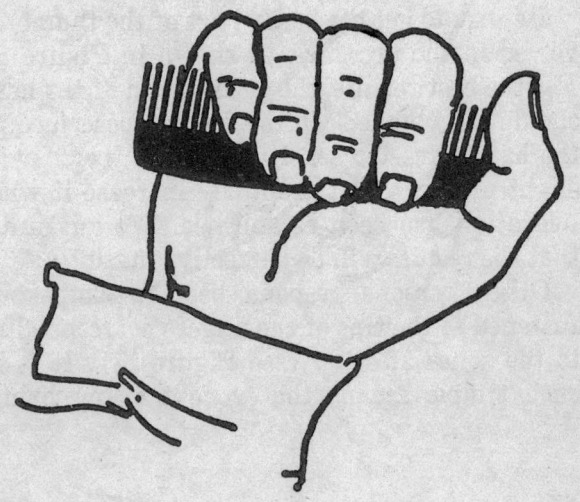

Figure 13.

Lumbago usually responds quite quickly to zone therapy, and cases of people doubled up with this sickness have been reported cured in one single treatment. Amazingly enough, the one tool that has been found the most beneficial is an ordinary aluminum comb, such as the kind that is used for dog-combing purposes (see Figure 13). The way to use it is to press the teeth of the comb against the inner surfaces of the fingers of each hand and, later, against the palms of the hands. For best results, such pressure must be maintained for ten or even twenty minutes. Persistent cases of lumbago may require workouts of the web between the thumb and first finger, and also the web between the first and second fingers of each hand.

Be sure to get the fleshy part of the thumb involved in the pressure, as shown in Figure 13. For the best results, the entire palm of the hand should be "combed" in the fashion described. If the hands are too sensitive at first, begin with slight pressure and gradually increase it when toleration has been established. We guarantee that the results will be perfectly amazing!

Other persons respond best to clothespins fastened to the tips of the fingers corresponding to the zones affected (see Figure 14). It is by such simple means that zone therapy brings

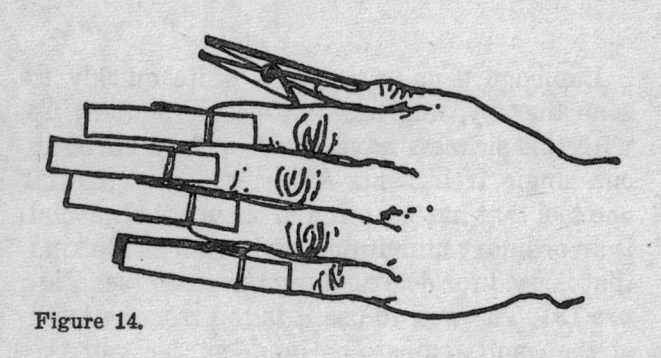

Figure 14.

lasting relief to the sufferings of the human body.

The clothespins may be left on for ten minutes at a time.

Proper massage of the lumbar region reflexes on the feet (see Figure 11) will bring relief to lumbago sufferers. You can be as thorough as tenderness permits.

9

Bladder Problems

Figure 15 will indicate with accuracy the reflex for the bladder. It lies in the lower lumbar region where the reflexes for the rectum and end of the spine are located, but not as deep as those two.

Cystitis, or inflammation of the bladder, is a fairly common disease causing a frequent desire to urinate. Fortunately, this is a condition which responds well to zone therapy on both feet. We recommend massage of the bladder reflex and the extension of this into the kidney reflex, because it is often the uric acid formed in the kidneys that causes the bladder to inflame (see Figure 16).

Press with your thumb into the soft part on the inside of the foot next to the heel pad. There you will find an area about the size of a quarter. Be sure to massage both feet in a similar fashion since we are dealing with zone one; the bladder lies in the middle of the body. Though the massage should be gentle, it should be persistent as well. If you are actually having trouble with your bladder, you should reach a point of pain,

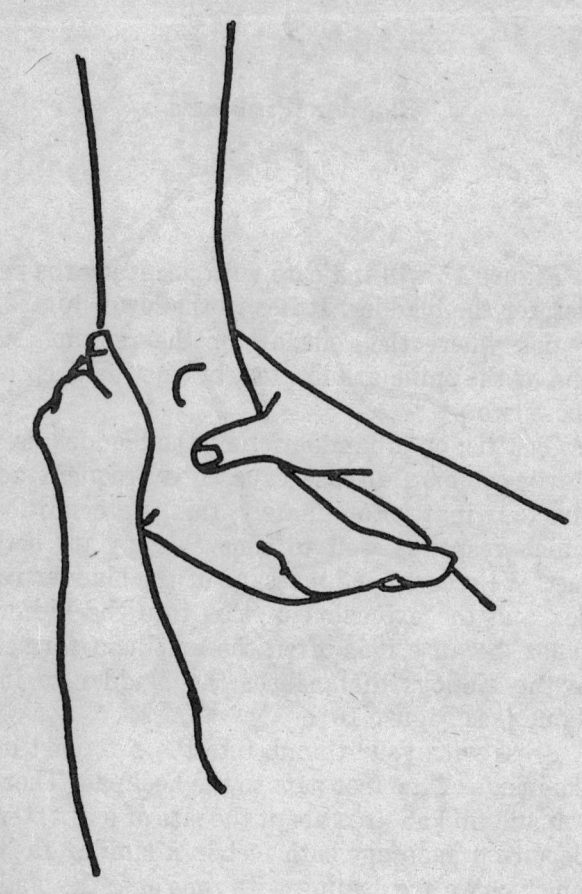

Figure 15.

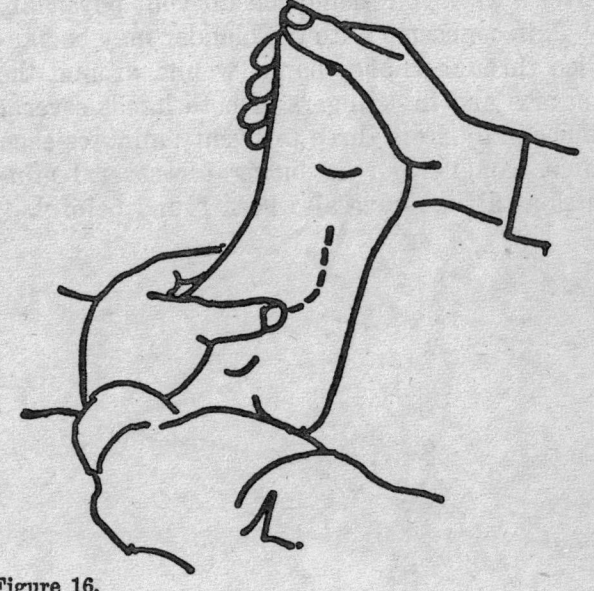

Figure 16.

which will be the bladder reflex. If not, continue to massage in a rotational way a little deeper until you find the spot.

It shouldn't take more than three treatments for a bladder condition to go away. But if there is blood in the urine or the condition persists after a week you should consult your physician.

Pain connected with the bladder may be handled through rubber bands wound around the thumbs and first fingers of both hands several times daily from three to twenty minutes each time. Tongue and lip biting for several minutes at a time have also been found helpful.

10

Blood Pressure

Blood pressure may be lowered by the application of rubber bands to the thumb and first and second fingers of both hands, and by massage of the webs between those fingers and between their joints.

On the other hand, blood pressure may be made to rise by rapidly stroking the entire body for several minutes, morning and night.

In any event, a physician should be consulted.

11

Colds, Sinusitis, Hay Fever

Who has not suffered through the ravages of a cold, emerging a week or so later looking pale and cadaverous? Colds are perhaps mankind's worst irritation, but not even twentieth-century science has been able to solve its riddle. Millions are spent on cold remedies that do little to alleviate the runny noses and sore throats associated with the common cold. So, if that is the case, why not try zone therapy?

There is as much controversy about colds as about how to run the government. Some believe colds are caused by germs attacking the respiratory system and that there is little that the average person can do about them. Others believe that if you take enough vitamin C you can avoid contagion. Still others say that colds are nature's way of cleaning house and eliminating an excess of toxic acid from the system. Be that as it may, we recommend that you suspend general massage of body reflexes and rest your feet, massaging only the toes and the reflexes for the lungs, followed by a short massage of the kidney reflex. Figure 16 shows where the kidneys are located; refer to Figure 4 for the lung reflexes.

The toes were mentioned above because these have to do directly with the sinuses. Congestion of the sinuses is one of the concomitant troubles that come with a bad cold, and congestion is one of the principal causes of trouble in any area. Fortunately, zone therapy works here where even medicines bring only partial relief.

The sinuses being in the head, we must attack the big toe. You should experience tenderness in various parts of the toes and there is where the massage should be applied. There will be a greater amount of pain along the base of the big toe, and you must press this area with two fingers coming from the inner and outer sides of the toe. Persist in this procedure, for the sinus condition won't surrender overnight.

Curiously enough, there is one spot between the second and third toes that appears to have a remarkable connection with the sinuses. If your sinuses are troubling you, experiment, because if you can locate the soreness in that area, a few minutes of massage can bring you relief as few medicines can.

Hay fever reacts to zone therapy treatments in almost all cases, and we urge sufferers of this irritating disorder to apply it to themselves as we shall indicate.

Although the causes of hay fever are as hazy as those for the cold, we know enough of its physical symptoms to state that it creates an acute inflammatory irritation in the nose. A vicious circle is formed whereby the irritation affects the nerves of the area, and these halt the circulation of the blood, causing still more pressure. In Dr. FitzGerald's treatise, he mentions finding a great number of his hay fever patients with somewhat abnormal nose conditions such as bony spurs, protruding turbinate bones, cartilage twisted out of alignment, and the like. He urged such persons to see specialists who could correct these physical conditions as a step toward the control of hay fever itself. He had good luck with applying firm pressure on various points on the roof of the mouth, and he used his thumb for this purpose. It is important to cover the region directly under the nose. The pressure should be maintained for from four to eight minutes at a time, and this should be repeated six or more times daily.

Doctors may want to bring relief to their patients by applying pressure with a cotton-tipped probe on the back wall of the pharynx, as well as directly on the mucous membranes of the nose. The probe may be dipped in trichloracetic acid for a more powerful "punch."

The layman will do well to attack a hay fever condition just as the sinus condition is attacked, by a workout of the reflexes on the big toes.

Other approaches may be tried; since every human being is different, not all approaches work the same, and it is wise to know several alternatives.

Relief has been found by simply pressing the upper lip against the teeth with the forefinger.

Also, a tongue depressor may be applied on the anterior half of the tongue several times a day. Biting the tongue and holding the bridge of the nose firmly between the thumb and forefinger also brings relief. Lastly, clothespins applied to the thumbs and first fingers should affect a hay fever condition.

12

Diabetes

If you will refer to Figure 9, you will see that the pancreas lies between the adrenal glands. Its reflex is a band that extends almost all the way across the left foot and a little over half way on the right foot. Diabetes is a condition brought on by the malfunctioning of the pancreas, so it is this organ that we wish to concentrate upon.

Whereas the reflex for the kidneys moves up the foot, the reflex for the pancreas runs across each foot, just above the kidney reflex. You may have some difficulty determining if you are on the right area, but the general rule applies: where you find soreness and tenderness, massage! (See Figure 17.)

Diabetics must be warned, however, that the reflex massage may induce an increase in the insulin supply, so it is best to discuss the fact that you intend to massage this area with your doctor, as it may be necessary to increase the intake of sugar.

If you work together with your doctor, the urine should be tested carefully during this

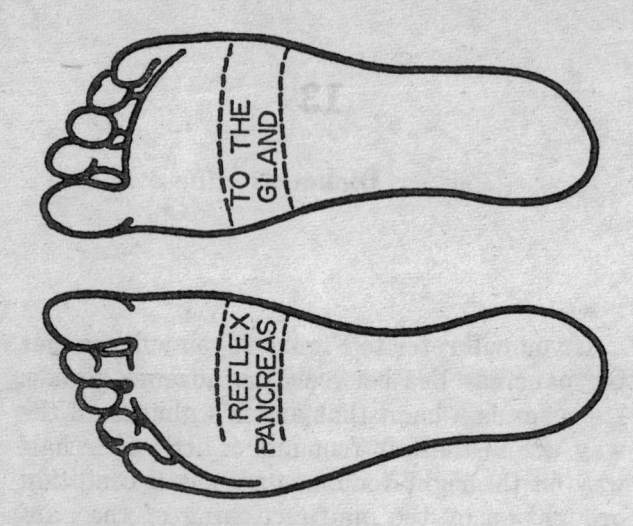

Figure 17.

period. It will be evident that massage in this area might force the liver to throw off some of its excess sugar into the system. If insulin is being used, you will want to continue its use until tests show that a lesser amount can be taken. Your physician will order the decrease, and will be happy to, inasmuch as the use of insulin is not a cure but merely a crutch to the system.

13

Ear Problems, Deafness

The ear is prone to many types of illnesses, so it should be obvious that not all approaches will work the same. This is also borne out by the fact that different parts of the ear involve different zones. We will list various approaches, one of which may just fit your condition and improve your hearing.

One of the handiest methods of curing hearing problems is to place a wad of absorbent lint in the space between the last tooth and the angle of the jaw, so that one is able to bite down hard. Formerly, some dentists would advise their patients to do just that with wonderful results. The "biting" should be prolonged for several minutes, two or three times a day.

Another method that has worked for some people is to squeeze the joints of the ring fingers or the toes corresponding to the ring fingers. There is little one can say to explain this from a scientific point of view, but it has worked where some of the world's greatest ear specialists have failed. In discussions that Dr. FitzGerald had with doctors familiar with zone therapy, he found that nine out of ten cases of otosclerosis or chronic congestion of the membranes of the ear could be improved from 25 to 90 percent following such crude methods.

Ringing of the ears and catarrhal deafness are also improved and sometimes cured by these approaches.

Some cases of deafness have been cured by pressing the teeth of an aluminum comb against the tips of the fingers of the hand (see Figure 18) five minutes at a time, and then following this up with pressure against the floor of the

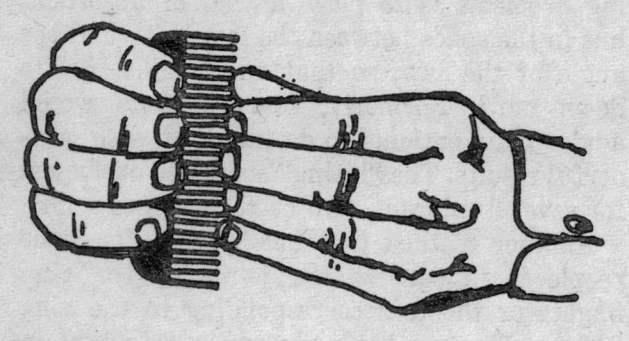

Figure 18.

mouth for six or seven minutes, then against the hard palate, and lastly against the tongue.

In cases of ear trouble, a very wise move is to have the wisdom teeth checked by a dentist. Often ear conditions develop due to a pathological condition of the back teeth.

One of the most effective earache cures we know is to fasten a clothespin for five minutes on the tip of the ring finger.

The most central reflex for the ears on the foot will be found in the area between the third and fourth toes and between the fourth and fifth toes. Tenderness in any such area should be massaged out for general relief of ear problems.

Hearing may generally be improved by the following procedure: Lift the end of the third fingernail of the right hand with the third fingernail of the left hand and do this forcibly for a few minutes at a time. Then do the same with the ring fingers. The same may be done with the middle and fourth toenails of both feet by using the fingernail of the index finger to do the lifting.

14

Epilepsy

Medical science still doesn't know what causes epilepsy; this illness is clouded in mystery, superstition, and even prejudice.

There are recorded cases of lessened epileptic attacks following zone therapy. A person suffering from epilepsy and willing to try zone therapy should experiment with his feet until he discovers areas of tenderness. In most cases, such a person will discover soreness under the big toe, where the reflex of the parathyroid gland is located. If so, proceed with caution, massaging for only a few minutes a day to determine if the attacks can be lessened.

Dr. FitzGerald's treatise speaks of dilatations from eight to ten minutes daily of mouth, nostrils, and external aural canals (packing the outer half of the canal tightly with cotton for a few minutes). He further suggests dilatation of the rectum, the vagina in women, and the urethra in men; for these procedures, medical attention should be sought.

15

Eye Problems

The reflexes to the eyes are found at the bottom of the second and third toes of each foot. It isn't difficult to massage these reflexes, and the way to do it is by a rolling motion done with two fingers. Press down and roll, searching for the sore spot that will indicate you have reached the trouble area, then massage it for a few seconds only.

Sometimes, abnormal eye conditions are caused by taut neck muscles that keep a good supply of blood from reaching the eyes. It is well to massage the top part of the feet, just where the second and third toes begin. The kidneys are also contributory factors in some ailments of the eye, so try massaging the kidney reflexes as well.

The main point of all this massaging is to bring back a healthy circulation of blood to the eyes. Cases of glaucoma have been reported improved by zone therapy; this tends to make sense, inasmuch as glaucoma is caused by the build-up of fluids which harden to produce partial or total blindness. A good blood supply just might inhibit this build-up, and zone therapy will activate circulation.

Eye strain may be relieved by tightly squeezing the knuckles of the first fingers of both hands. With persons whose eyes are especially set apart, this must be repeated on the middle fingers. Apply the pressure on the upper and lower surfaces as well as on the sides. Do this for five minutes at a time.

Sties and such conditions as conjunctivitis and granulated lids are completely relieved by pressure exerted upon the joints of the first and second fingers of the hand corresponding to the diseased eye. Sties can be cleared up in one or two treatments; with other inflammatory conditions, it is necessary to persist for several weeks, treating the eyes to zone therapy three times each week.

Dr. FitzGerald mentions curing patients of inflammation of the optic nerve—a condition which leads to blindness. He did this by applying pressure on the fingers as mentioned and following this by applying pressure with a probe over the inferior dental nerve, where it enters the lower jaw bone; doctors, take notice.

Dr. FitzGerald gives further advice to physicians as follows: "I should like to add that in treating eye strain, conjunctivitis, sties, granulated lids, and eye conditions generally, pressures made with a blunt probe on the mucocutaneous margins (where the skin joins the mucous membrane in the nostrils) affects the second division of the ophthalmic nerve, and assists materially in bringing about a favorable influence in eye troubles.

"I would also emphasize the importance of seeing that the condition of the eye teeth was perfect, as frequently some chronic inflammatory eye trouble may be caused by an infection from the roots of the canine teeth."

We'd like to sum up by saying that any condition of the eyes brought on by an excess of nerve or muscle tension or faulty circulation can be taken care of by the squeezing of the fingers described earlier. As Dr. FitzGerald put it: "If you don't believe it, try it. It costs nothing but a few minutes' intelligent effort."

16

Fatigue and Depression

Everyone has gone through periods where it seemed impossible to get through the day. Indeed, fatigue is the almost constant companion of large numbers of people in this age of anxiety. People, too, cause their own troubles, by crowding their time with all kinds of activities until they have no time to relax and rest.

Refer to Figure 9. There you will see the reflexes for the all-important glands that should be massaged if you wish to be rid of that feeling of exhaustion. Begin with the most important gland of all, the pituitary, by giving the center of your toe a quick massage, pressing deeply enough to affect this gland. Continue with a massage of the thyroid reflex, and then move on to the adrenal reflexes. Half a minute there will be enough for the pickup you are looking for. After that, tackle the reflex of the sex glands, or gonads, situated in your ankle. No more than fifteen seconds are required for these glands, after which you repeat this procedure on the other foot.

As a final step, you may want to massage the

spleen, producer of red blood cells. This involves the left foot only (see Figure 4). Do it for half a minute and then go back to the pituitary gland reflex and give it a final deep massage of a few seconds' duration. You will notice the difference immediately in your well-being and actual pep.

Depression is closely connected with body fatigue, although we tend to think of it as exclusively mental. The point is that we wouldn't feel depression if our bodily health was up to par. Depression, then, is tied in with fatigue of long duration. To cure it, we suggest the previous massage and, in addition, some attention paid to the pineal gland reflex, which is also located on the big toe. Massage that area as well, since the pineal gland is believed to have a lot to do with organizing the functioning of the endocrine glands.

Continuing mental depression is a sign of psychic problems, and a person suffering from this should seek proper medical attention.

17

Childbirth, Morning Sickness, Menopause, Menstrual Cramps

Women suffer from a wide variety of problems, and it takes a practiced therapist to discover their source. Conditions in many parts of the body may affect the proper functioning of the female organs. Often, the cause of many a trouble is the tension and tightening up of the muscles of the uterus and vagina, and the concomitant nervousness that this will produce.

Trouble with the ovaries can sometimes be traced to a malfunctioning thyroid gland, considered by some as a third ovary. Massage of the thyroid reflex as well as the ovary reflexes will correct such conditions (see Figure 19 for ovary reflex).

On the other hand, if there is hemorrhage, do not use any massage; consult your physician.

Certain functions of the ovaries (and the testes in men) are related to the pituitary gland. They have far-reaching functions in the body and are not connected exclusively with reproductive functions.

The massage of the area above the soles of the feet and under the ankle bone stimulates

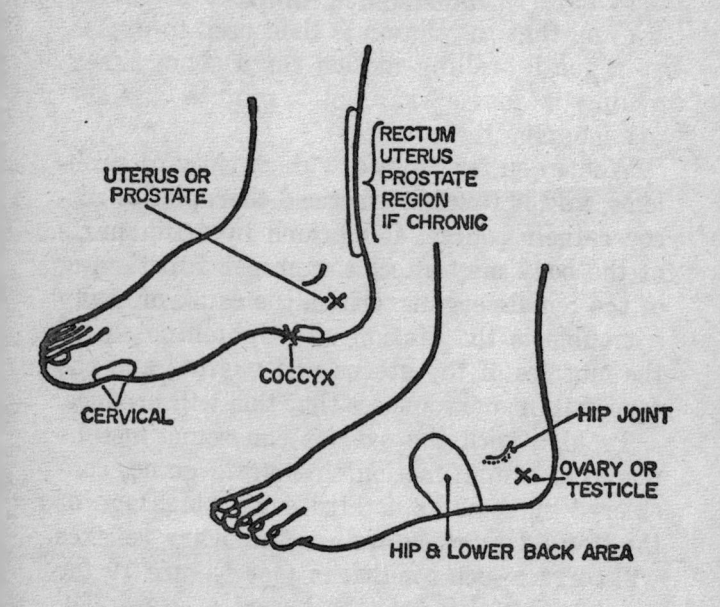

SAME REFLEX AREAS FOUND ON BOTH FEET

Figure 19.

the ovaries, uterus, and fallopian tubes in the female, and the testicles, penis, and prostate gland in the male. Inflammation in the sex organ areas will show up in tenderness where these reflexes lie. Figure 20 shows how best to massage this area. Notice that the foot is pulled back and that the thumb is then used to press. Use a gentle, rolling motion for a short time, certainly no longer than half a minute, and always massage the two feet.

The pains of childbirth can be relieved, and the process of labor accelerated by six hours, through zone therapy. The method is simplicity itself; it consists of clasping an aluminum

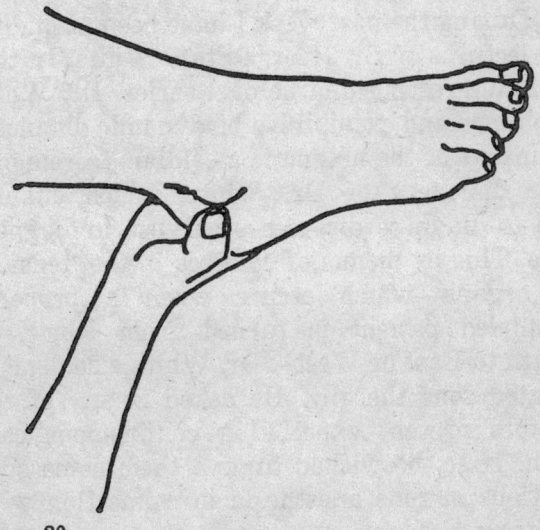

Figure 20.

85

comb in each hand, as in Figure 13, and holding tight intermittently from the time the contractions begin until delivery. In addition, the soles of the feet should be pressed against some edged surface (a wire brush will do). Rubber bands wound around the big toes and next toes also bring relief.

After-pains are relieved and the expulsion of the after birth is facilitated by stroking the reflex zones in the hands, arms, and legs with an aluminum comb or a wire brush from every ten minutes to half an hour. These assist in the contraction of the uterus.

We must quote a passage from Dr. Fitz-Gerald. He quotes a Dr. R. T. H. Nesbitt, of Waukegan, Illinois, who sent him the following report:

"During the past week I have been attending the lectures of Dr. George Starr White. In this most interesting and helpful series, Dr. White explained and exemplified biodynamic diagnosis by means of the magnetic meridian (a remarkable discovery of Dr. White, which enables one to diagnose diseases otherwise undiagnosable. This by means of changes in the 'tension' of organs—which occurs when a properly grounded patient is turned from North or South to East or West). Dr. White also demonstrated zone therapy. He asked if any of the doctors present expected a confinement case soon. If so, he wished to give them some suggestions in zone anesthesia in connection with delivery.

"As I was expecting a call ever hour I told Dr. White, and he gave me some special points concerning this work. Last night I was called to attend what I expected would be my last case in confinement, as I have been doing this work so many years that I intended to retire. From my last night's experience I feel as if I should like to start the practice of medicine all over again.

"The woman I delivered was a primipara (one who had never had a child before, and who, therefore, because of the rigidity of the bones and tissues, has a more difficult labor), small in stature.

"When severe contractions began, and the mother was beginning to be very nervous and complained of pain, at which time I generally administer chloroform, I began pressing on the soles of the feet with the edge of a big file, as I could find nothing else. I pressed on the top of the foot with the thumbs of both hands at the metatarsal-phalangeal joint (where the toes join the foot). I exerted this pressure over each foot for about three minutes at a time. The mother told me that the pressure on the feet gave her no pain whatsoever.

"As she did not have any uterine pain, I was afraid there was no advancement. To my great surprise, when I examined her about ten or fifteen minutes later, I found the head within two inches of the outlet. I then waited about fifteen minutes, and on examination found the head at the vulva. I then pressed again for about one or two minutes on each foot, the edge of the file being on the sole of the foot, and my thumbs over the tarsal-metatarsal joints as before. In this way I exerted pressure on the sole of the foot with the file, and pressure on the dorsum of the foot with my thumbs, doing each foot separately. The last pressure lasted about one and a half minutes on each foot. Within five or ten minutes the head was appearing, and I held it back to preserve the perineum (the tissue joining the vagina and the rectum). It made steady progress, the head and shoulders coming out in a normal manner. Within three minutes the child —which weighed in at 9½ pounds—was born, crying lustily. The mother told me she did not experience any pain whatever, and could not believe the child was born. She laughed and said, 'This is not so bad.'

"Another point that is very remarkable is that after the child was born the woman did not experience the fatigue that is generally felt, and the child was more active than usual. I account for this on the principle that pain inhibits progress of the birth, and tires the child. But as the pain was inhibited, the progress was more steady, and thus fatigue to both mother and child was avoided."

Other equally remarkable cases of painless chilbirth could be given. Aluminum combs to hold in the hands have been tried with success; at such times, a rough-edged box should be placed in the bed so that the patient may be able to press against it with her feet.

Cases of morning sickness may be cured by the use of rubber bands applied on the thumbs and index fingers and by applying pressure on the webs between these fingers.

Hot flashes play an important part in the history of menopause. Women age more rapidly then, and they tend to suffer from insomnia and nervousness. These symptoms can be alleviated by the proper massage of the ovary reflexes, since these will control production of the hormone estrogen. In connection with the massage of the ovary reflexes, there should also be massage of the pituitary gland reflex. Such a practice will enable a woman to go through menopause in a smoother fashion.

Painful menstruation yields like magic to the pressure of a probe aimed at the back wall of the pharynx, but again, we do not recommend that anyone but a physician carry this out. On the other hand, tongue biting is sometimes effective.

For pain in the back or in the thighs, preceding or during menstruation, pressure with the index finger on the back wall of the pharynx will give relief. Also, a tongue depressor may be used to press down on the tongue about three quarters of the way back. This should be done with the help of another person who can hold the patient's head rigid and support the lower jaw. This way the proper amount of pressure

—which should be strong—can be applied. It should last for two minutes, then relaxed and the point of focus changed slightly. Many women who were formerly obliged to go to bed for two or three days each month have been relieved of all distress after a course of this treatment.

Please note that tongue pressure should not be applied in the case of pregnancy.

Lastly, we must note that pressure brought to bear on the thumbs and the first and second fingers of both hands can bring relief of menstrual cramps. Use fingers or clothespins.

18

Gallbladder

Figure 21 indicates where the gallbladder reflex is located. Actually, the gallbladder reflex proper is a bit below and more toward the center of the liver reflex. A little experience will tell you where it is, but you should proceed with caution. Too much massage of the liver reflex can make you quite sick for a while, since it may release a lot of stored-up poisons. It is best to proceed with caution, and massage only a few seconds at a time at first.

The gallbladder is lodged under the right lobe of the liver and is the body's receptacle for bile. It is also the place where gallstones can congregate.

Any tenderness in this area should be massaged carefully. Don't try to massage all the tenderness out in the first try. Zone therapy has helped dissolve gallstone and thus averted painful operations, but it is best not to rush the job.

We do not know if massage of the gallbladder actually dissolves gallstone or simply allows

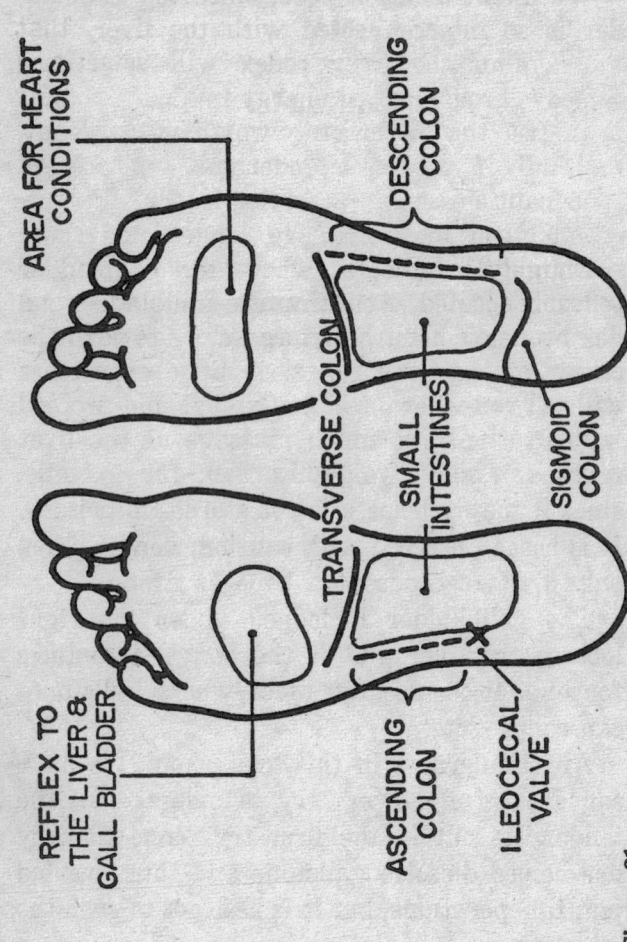

Figure 21.

their passage through and out, but it certainly does something to alleviate the condition.

We might mention here, since the gallbladder is so interconnected with the liver, that massage of the liver reflex will sometimes remedy chronic lack of energy in a person. This is an area that is certainly worth checking out, especially if you detect tenderness. Just proceed with caution. After a while, if the liver responds, you may massage longer and more thoroughly.

Rubber bands on the thumbs, first and second fingers, and comparable toes will have a beneficial effect on the gallbladder and may be tried without fear of a liver reaction.

19

Goiter

Goiter used to be quite a prevalent condition, although it seemed to vary from place to place, some areas being more conducive to it than others. Nowadays, a great deal more is known about the thyroid gland and the use of iodine in the system, so enlargement of the thyroid is rare.

In the first part of this century, when Dr. Fitzgerald was writing and working, goiters were a bothersome malady, but he had learned how to deal with them thanks to zone therapy; he did so by the use of probes passed through the nostrils and applied to the back wall of the pharynx. He also insisted on placing rubber bands around the thumb, first and second fingers, and sometimes even the ring finger, keeping them there for ten or fifteen minutes at a time three or four times daily.

20

Headaches, Migraine

Instead of using aspirin and other highly touted pills for headaches—which are taken by the millions, with unimaginable after-effects—people should follow zone therapy for relief, for nothing could be simpler and less harmful.

If the headache is due to neuralgia or nervous strain, the best remedy is to press your thumb or something like a spoon against the roof of the mouth, as nearly as possible under the part that hurts. The pressure should be maintained for from three to five minutes, no less. If the headache is extensive, you may have to shift the pressure to cover the rest of the roof of the mouth.

These points of pressure may extend from the roots of the front teeth, for a frontal headache, to the junction of the soft and hard palates when the headache lies in the back of the head. Likewise, from one side of the mouth to the other if the headache is located to one side of the head.

If the headache is caused by other conditions, the case gets a little more complicated. For instance, there are headaches caused by poisons caused by improper bowel movements, constipation, too many drinks the night before, or eye-strain. Little help will be obtained from the above method in these cases.

On the other hand, headaches frequently respond to pressure exerted over the joints of the thumb or fingers. Dr. White once cured a woman patient who had suffered from a headache for three weeks by firmly pressing the first, second, and third fingers of her hands.

The best approach when a headache is due to eye-strain is to relax the neck area by massaging the entire big toe in the following manner: Take it between two fingers and rotate it right and left, round and round until relief comes.

If you know that a specific organ is causing your headache (the stomach or liver, for example), work the big toe as indicated and then work on the reflex to that organ.

Many other headaches are cured by massaging the connecting spot between the big toe and the next toe. You might notice a tenderness there, or might search for it, because some headaches don't give up unless that zone is massaged. Even migraine will yield to the right spot between the toes. Look for it, for in some people it may be located between two other toes!

21

Heart Disorders

Heart failure can be prevented through zone therapy, and we would like to discuss this now at some length. No one will argue the fact that the heart is one of the most important organs in the body; it is a strong muscle, capable of working night and day for a lifetime without presenting its owner with the least bit of trouble. But we tend to take advantage of a good thing; we abuse it and then wonder why it gives us trouble. Zone therapy can tell you just how much you have been leaning on your heart, and it is important that you learn to work the heart reflex so that you can engage in the proper preventive measures. See Figure 22 for the right way to massage this all-important reflex. You will notice how the thumb presses in on the pad of the little toe. The heart is not that small an organ, so you may massage the area with some degree of certainty. Any tenderness there is an indication of some degree of congestion, which, if allowed to continue unchecked for some time, could lead to heart attack.

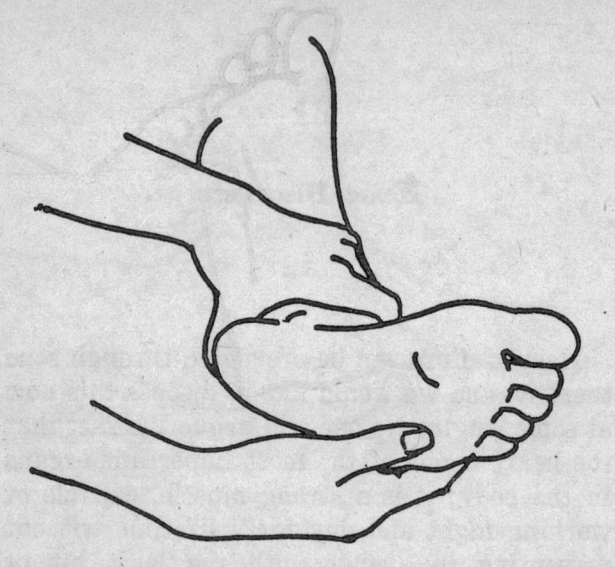

Figure 22.

The heart and the muscles directly connected to it are located slightly to the left of the chest cavity, so that the reflex to this all-important organ is to be found in the second, third, and fourth zones of the left foot (see Figure 23 for correct position for massaging the heart reflex).

Tenderness in this area may be an indication of congestion and this could lead, in the long run, to a heart attack. Now since the heart is well buried in the chest cavity, it will be necessary for you to apply strong pressure to reach the right reflex. Use the front of the thumb, and the nail as well.

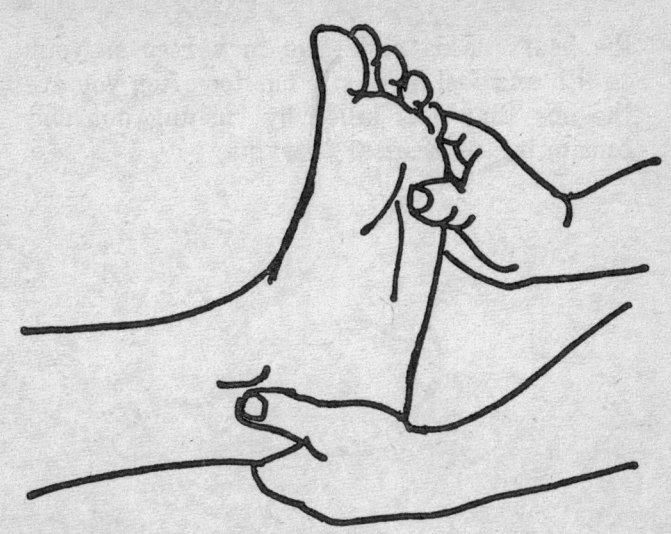

Figure 23.

No matter what your trouble may be, you can aid your heart through zone therapy. Sometimes, massaging the heart reflex will lead to a sensation of pain shooting from the foot to the heart, but this is followed by a good feeling and it means that the heart has been aided.

With angina pectoris, where pains shoot up the shoulder and arm, you must work over a wide area of reflexes, from the base of the little toe and the third and fourth toes down to the center of the heart reflex. The shoulder pains may be aided by massaging the little toe itself.

One note of warning must be uttered. Sometimes if the pains disappear, a person is apt to take up where he left off. But remember that the heart needs rest. You may recover your health and feel fit to kill, but too often you are the one that gets killed by rushing out and continuing unnecessary strains.

22

Hemorrhoids

Hemorrhoids are those extremely painful veins that have become congested and protrude from the rectum. Not only are they a great inconvenience, but they sometimes bleed and require surgical care.

Zone therapy can work wonders with hemorrhoids, dissipating the pain that accompanies them. Apply yourself to their reflexes as shown in Figure 23. Here is how to do it: Instead of a rolling type of massage, press in towards the bone and down towards the heel, firmly. Do this all the way around the heel, using the thumb for one side and the index finger for the other. Be sure to apply plenty of pressure and do this on both feet. Recheck for specific sore spots and massage those a little longer than the rest of the reflex. At first you may have trouble in finding any soreness whatever, but that is because you may not be pressing hard enough. Move the flesh of the heel back and forth against the bone until you find the tenderness; if you suffer from hemorrhoids, it will be there.

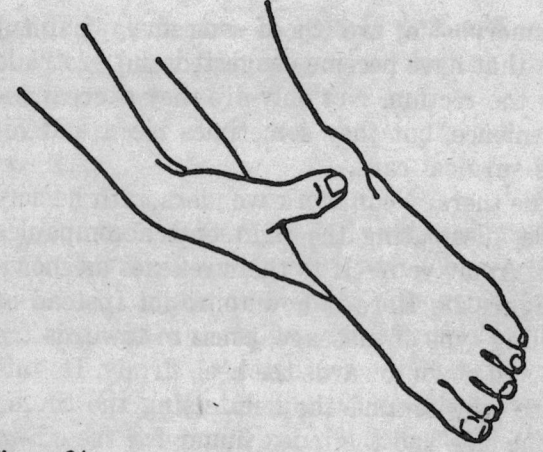

Figure 24.

23

Hiccoughs

The founding fathers of zone therapy found several marvelous ways to deal with this little malady. Dr. FitzGerald, in his usual charming manner, describes one method as follows: "For, when we grasp the tongue of the hiccougher, and with a long pull, a strong pull, and a pull all together, haul the offending member to tongue's length—and hold it there—we cure the spasmodic contraction of the diaphragm (the cause of the hiccough) by influencing the zone in which the trouble originates."

Other methods include interlocking all the fingers of the hands firmly and holding them there, exerting as much pressure as possible; applying clothespins to the tips of the thumbs and fingers; and, lastly, applying pressure on the tongue with a tongue depressor, right in the middle. Good luck!

24

Infections, Lymph Glands, Kidneys

Infections can occur anywhere on the body if the skin has been broken and foreign objects have penetrated. It is a good idea to keep the lymph glands in shape by massaging their reflex in the feet, for it is the lymph glands that take the main burden of fighting infection throughout the body.

These lymph glands compose an entire network of vessels that collect fluids seeping through the walls of blood vessels. This material collects at specific nodes in the armpits, in the groin, and all around the neck. It is calculated that there are between six and seven hundred nodes in the body. Figure 25 indicates their location as a reflex in the foot, and the way to message this reflex.

The whole area on top of the foot should be massaged, from one side of the ankle bone to the other. Use as many fingers as you find convenient, or the whole of the thumb, pressing and circling. Be sure to massage both feet.

If you will refer to Figure 11 you will see just where the kidney reflexes are located.

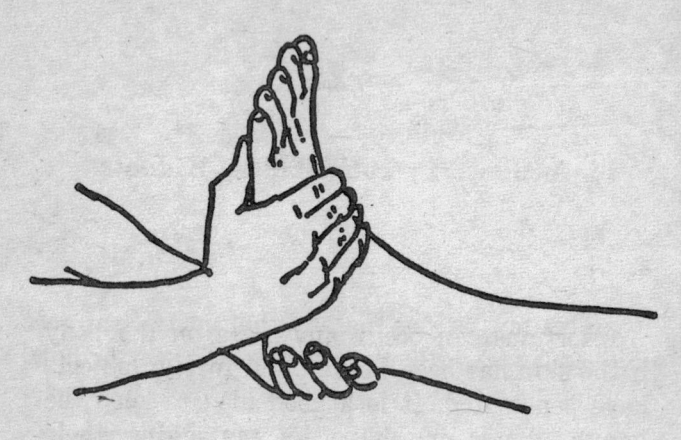

Figure 25.

Since the kidneys have the job of ridding the entire organism of accumulated poisons, normal and abnormal, you will understand why we suggest that you go easy on them at first. There can be such a thing as overmassaging the kidney reflexes at the beginning, when they are not used to it and are overloaded with poisons. If the reflexes are tender, proceed slowly and do not massage more than a minute each day for the first few days.

As we have already mentioned, the kidneys may affect the eyes, so in cases of eye-strain, try massaging the kidney reflexes.

Severe infections should logically involve massage of the lymph gland reflexes and the kidney reflexes as well.

25

Insomnia

This mysterious malady that comes and goes like a curse, without your knowing why or how, can be controlled by one of several methods, all vouched for by Dr. FitzGerald and Dr. Bowers.

The first approach is to interlock all the fingers of the two hands for no less than ten minutes, pressing as hard as you can stand it.

The second method is to stroke your forearms on all their surfaces with a wire brush, or, if no wire brush is available, with your fingernails. This is to be carried on for five or ten minutes.

Lastly, you may press with your thumb and index finger above the bridge of the nose, holding that position for ten minutes.

26

Joint Pains

Sometimes we wake up in the morning with vague pains across the back of the neck and shoulders. The best way to relieve this kind of tension is to press strongly with the knuckles of your hand against the sole of the foot, while with the fingers of the other hand you dig in and try to loosen the ligaments and muscles across the top of the foot directly above the area you are working with your knuckles.

Body joints will tend to ache where there is any tendency to broken metatarsal arches. Our advice is to see a foot specialist who will recommend the right kind of shoes to buy in order to correct this condition. The difference this will make in your everyday energy is astounding.

Leg cramps can be disposed of by the simple expedient of massaging the cords in back of the knee. Try that next time you are semi-paralyzed from a cramp.

Remember that in zone therapy the knee corresponds with the elbow, and the hip with the shoulder of the same side. Firm manipulation of the joints of the thumbs, fingers, hand, elbow, and shoulder affect positively the corresponding joints in the lower extremity. You may pull, flex, extend, and rotate the various parts at the same time that you apply pressure, holding various positions for a few seconds.

After you have treated the hand or wrist, compare it with the other hand and wrist for lightness and flexibility and then see if you notice any difference in the feet. It may take you a while to catch these differences, but the connections are surely there.

If you treat these zones this way you may find yourself rid of aches and pains, and much relaxed.

27

Nervousness

Nervousness is a condition endemic to contemporary living, and of course different people deal with it in different ways. You can take pills, tranquilizers, and thus function. Or, if you have the money, you can go to a psychiatrist and go into the problem at length.

Zone therapy cannot help you if the causes are psychic disturbances, but for that occasional feeling of butterflies in your stomach or a particularly difficult period of adjustment to a new job or a new mate, here are some simple, workable methods of reducing tension:

From a preventive point of view, you might try the ten minute daily toning-up exercises listed in the last chapter of this book. However, if you are presently in the throes of a nervous attack, try placing rubber bands on the first, second, and third fingers of both hands and, if that is not enough, on the respective toes as well.

Clenching of the hands for prolonged periods is extremely relaxing and is highly recommended for the nervous system; it should be done while the jaws are firmly set against each other. The interlocking of the fingers of both hands is another method that works just as well, and is something that we do instinctively in times of stress or shock, when emotions are at their peak.

The best suggestion is to take a wire brush and brush the entire body with it, from the fingertips to the tips of the toes. Do it for five minutes in the morning and then again before retiring for the night.

Some people, in manifesting extreme anger, will bite their lip, sometimes hard enough to bleed. The majority, as we have said, will clench their hands and double up their toes in their shoes. Nobody has come up with a reason for it, but we do it and will continue to do it involuntarily and automatically because such actions relieve pain and nervous tension. They produce an actual form of analgesia similar to that which follows the injection of an anesthetic into a sensory nerve.

So people who scoff at zone therapy are not paying attention to what the body itself is telling them. Dr. FitzGerald certainly believed in it, and was patient enough to work at it for several months in some cases. He cites the case of a woman with writer's cramp caused by her nervousness. She suffered so much from it that she couldn't hold a pen and was unable to sleep at night. It took him months to cure her, but he did it. And it was done by using an aluminum comb and combing the front and back of her hands and her fingertips, and pressing her tongue down with a tongue depressor for four or five minutes a day.

28

Neuralgia

Reference to Figures 6 and 7 should tell you in which zone the pain lies and will therefore guide you as to how best to attack the condition through the feet reflexes. Most often, neuralgia will yield to pressure on thumbs, fingers, or toes of the zones involved, but we suggest that a doctor be consulted in the event that there is an infection of the teeth or something similar.

Dr. FitzGerald also suggests packing the outer third of the aural canal tightly with slightly moistened cotton.

He mentions a case of another doctor friend of his, Dr. Roemer, who treated a patient with trifacial neuralgia of two years' standing. Nothing had helped this man; his attacks were often of four and five days' duration, at which times he was unable to speak. Speech brought him paroxysms of pain that radiated over the entire left side of his face, from the lower to the upper jaw and up into the left eye, leaving him limp as a rag.

Dr. Roemer applied rubber bands on the joints nearest the tip of the thumb and forefinger of the left hand. In less than ten minutes the patient was talking and laughing. His advice to the man was to apply the bands for half an hour if another attack came on.

29

Neuritis

Neuritis can be extremely painful and crippling. Cases of neuritis of the shoulder, for instance, are reported after a person has suffered a hard fall and injured that extremity. Bones may not be broken, but the nerves are neverthelesss affected and, in due time, pain builds and builds until it is so severe that the person cannot move the limb at all.

Obviously, in a condition such as that, you must find the reflex area in the foot and go to work, carefully at first since the pain in the foot will be intense! It is best to work for a minute or two and then rest, but a twenty-minute workout would not be too unusual if you want to make progress. In cases of shoulder problems you will work below the little toe. It might take as long as a week but results will come (see Figure 24).

Dr. FitzGerald cured a man suffering from neuritis of the arm and shoulder for six years by clamping clothespins on the fingers of the affected arm for twelve minutes, after which the man was able to raise his arm over his head for the first time. Following a few weeks' treatment of five-minute applications of tight rubber bands around the ends of his fingers, the man reported himself cured.

Sciatic neuritis can be helped with deep pressure from the teeth of an aluminum comb upon the toes.

30

Paralysis, Strokes

Apoplexy, or the type of stroke caused by a blood clot in the brain, is in turn caused by a hemorrhage somewhere in the brain. It usually affects one side of the body, the side opposite to where the clot in the brain is located. The paralysis may be complete or partial.

The paralysis is brought about by the pressure which the clot brings to bear on that part of the brain controlling the motor action of the part of the body paralyzed. The nervous impulses governing action cannot be transmitted and thus the muscles cannot move.

Paralysis may or may not be incurable, depending on the location of the clot, its size, the health of the individual, and the capacity of the organism to begin absorbing the clot. If the clot begins to be absorbed, it will allow the brain to once again begin transmitting messages through to the afflicted part.

How can zone therapy work in a case like this? It pays to go back and realize that the cause of this paralysis is more often than not high blood pressure. That is the real culprit, so it behooves us to check and see if the kidneys, liver, and other organs are doing their part the way they should. This should not be difficult once you understand foot reflexes and how they respond. For whatever is really behind this condition will respond with marked tenderness. This is the first step, and it might take some time to remove the cause of it. But it makes sense, doesn't it, that by removing the obstacles in the way of proper blood circulation you are doing for your body what it really needs done to get on the road to health.

To assist the brain directly to get over the condition, you must tackle the brain reflexes in the big toe. Some of the reflexes cross behind the neck, so that if the right side of the body has been paralyzed we must work on the toe of the left foot. If any part of this toe is tender, massage it out, thus assisting the circulation of blood in the brain. It won't hurt to massage the toe on the side afflicted as well, to benefit the entire brain.

31

Pneumonia

Nobody plays with pneumonia; it is a very serious condition in which the lungs or the bronchial tubes are acutely inflamed due to either a virus, bacterial attack, or other causes such as aspiration of foreign material into the lungs. The first thing that zone therapy can do is alleviate the congestion and relieve tension by massaging the reflexes for shoulders and lungs.

Dr. FitzGerald was keen on rubber bands on all fingers or toes or on both, plus tongue pressure with tongue depressor and the use of a cotton-tipped probe on appropriate zones of the mouth, pharynx, and nose.

Reflex massage of the lung areas in both feet will benefit the bronchial tubes, but bear in mind that the massage should be deep. Start under the big toe, in the same place where the throat reflexes are located, so you cover the entire respiratory apparatus. Press in with the thumb into the soft area under the toe and massage all the way down to the end of the pad, moving with a pressing yet circular motion.

With fever, be sure to cover the pituitary gland reflex as well.

32

Prostate Problems

The prostate gland lies directly in front of the rectum, so the reflexes will be the same for the prostate and the rectum. The prostate is the largest male sex gland, and it circles the neck of the urethra as it emerges from the bladder. Its location, for our purposes, is in the first zone of both feet.

An enlargement of this gland—that is, any amount of congestion—will cause great pain and inconvenience when it comes to voiding urine. As it also affects the nervous system, it is important to keep it functioning properly.

Any indisposition of this gland will result in the reflex being quite tender, perhaps extending down to the lower portion of the inside of the heel, in the direction of the bladder reflex (see Figure 26).

Fortunately, zone therapy can get this gland back to health in a relatively short time. Note the position of the hand (Figure 27) in massaging this area, and how the thumb presses one side above the heel while the knuckle of the forefinger presses from the other side, aided

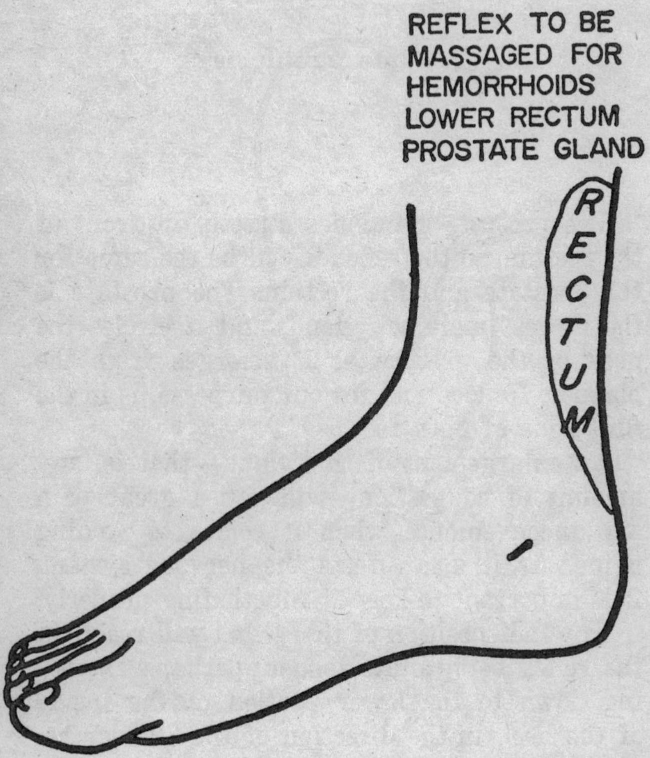

Figure 26.

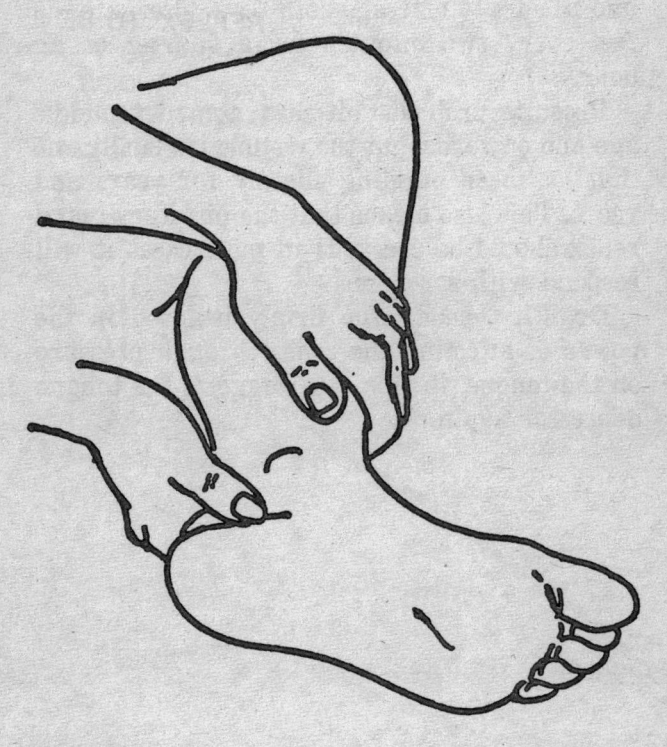

Figure 27.

by the rest of the fingers for additional strength. The actual reflex is about half an inch in from the cord going up the back of the leg. Try a pressing, rolling type of rotation, and be sure to massage both feet. Alternate the feet every two minutes for a quarter of an hour.

Prostate problems hit men at about middle age and onwards, but the trouble is usually one that has been building silently for years and years. This also means that the pituitary gland reflex should be checked; in most cases it will respond with soreness.

Dr. FitzGerald, who firmly believed in the power of affecting the zones through pressure on the tongue, in this case suggests the tongue depressor again.

33

Rectum Disorders, Prolapsed Rectum

We have seen that the reflex to the rectum, prostate, and hemorrhoids is one and the same, with hemorrhoids logically at the heel.

Rectal problems may be large or small. If large, they may extend, as far as reflexology is concerned, as far as three to four inches up from the heel. Proceed as with the massage for bladder problems, bending the foot back as far as possible, stretching the cord immediately beneath the skin and tackling the flesh to the inside of it. When you have worked out some of the tenderness from the area, go back and massage the cord itself. It may be agony because the inflammation of the rectum will have provided its reflex with enough tenderness for the massage to be anything but fun, but grit your teeth and bear down because the results will pay big dividends.

Often, as a person gets older, a condition known as a prolapsus or prolapsed rectum sets in. This is nothing but the gradual and very painful and uncomfortable protruding of the rectum, and it is usually accompanied by its acute inflammation and swollen condition. Apply here the same approach as for hemorrhoids; the results will no doubt amaze you!

34

Relaxation

Interlocking the fingers of the hand and squeezing for all you are worth is about the oldest and best way there is to relax, if you can manage to do it for more than a few minutes at a time. If you are serious about it, however, and do just what we tell you, you will discover that no matter how rough and rotten a day you have had, a soothing feeling will steal all over your body and your cares will seem to dissolve in consequence. If you tire of the first approach, you may switch to applying firm pressure on finger and thumb tips. Clothespins are marvelous for this therapy because once you have applied them you can forget them and even take a nap. You will awaken a different person!

Another approach, mentioned before, is the setting of the jaws by biting down hard and keeping the pressure constant. This may be facilitated by taking a piece of rubber or cloth and biting on it instead. If there is no one around to make fun of you while you're at it, try stretching your lips outward, for as many minutes as you can stand it. It works!

35

Rheumatism

First off, we might mention that rheumatism is one of those mysterious ailments that science hasn't gotten around to solving yet. It attacks thousands and thousands of people and there is very little that they can do ... unless they know zone therapy.

Dr. FitzGerald had a hunch, which he set down for whatever it was worth, that offending corns, warts, and bitten fingernails may be responsible for rheumatic conditions. Is that the case with you? Does your rheumatism go hand in hand with any of those little-suspected happenings?

He mentions a peculiar case of his in which a patient, suffering from rheumatism of the left shoulder and arm, had been unable to sleep for more than three weeks on account of the pain. But he had a small callus on the tip of his left thumb that corresponded to the zone where his pain was located. When the callus was removed and pressure with a comb applied to the area, the man was cured within four days!

Rheumatism responds to zone therapy. Treat the zones involved and the pain will begin to disappear. Apply rather hard massage twice a day to the zone involved, on both feet or one as the case may be.

36

Sciatica

The old medical sages of zone therapy suggested, first off, that you look for an infection in the mouth or elsewhere, holding that the third molar teeth were often responsible.

One of the key sensitive areas in sciatica, in the hand, is the junction of hand and wrist, in the palmar surface. Press tightly with an aluminum comb.

Sciatic neuritis has been cured with deep pressure by an aluminum comb on the fleshy part of the toes as well as on the fingers. If the pain is severe in the back of the legs, use the comb to apply pressure on the sole of the foot. If the pain occurs in the front part of the legs, the top of the foot should be pressed with the comb. However, the best and most rapid relief for sciatica is obtained by attacking the soles of the feet. In fact, Dr. White even "invented" a device consisting of a piece of hard wood about five inches in length cut with deep screw-like threads. He had a hole drilled through it and a rope inserted, so that the patient could use it with a strong pull for five and ten minutes at a time, several times a day.

If sciatica is due to hip dislocation, zone therapy may not be as favorable. A twisting of the hip or subluxation of the hip joint may be a condition best treated by your doctor or chiropractor. But try zone therapy first!

Look at it this way: The sciatic nerve is the biggest nerve in the body, three-quarters of an inch wide. Coming out of the pelvis, it descends along the back of the thigh and later divides into two. If this big nerve ever gets inflamed, you are obviously in for a lot of pain. And the causes may be many, not just your dislocated hip. It may be due to an injury sustained in quite another part of the body, to an inflamed prostate gland, to constipation, or to a misplacement of the vertebra. Look at Figure 28 for the proper way to massage the reflex to this important nerve and try using the eraser end of a good pencil.

The reason for the pencil is that this is a deeply buried reflex and only a fairly sharp instrument is going to reach it. Please notice that the reflex will be found back from the center of the heel pad, toward the outside of the foot.

Massage with a deep, rolling action, doing your best to forget the intense pain that it might bring if the right spot has been located. There have been people who have found a cure for their pain in one or two treatments, but

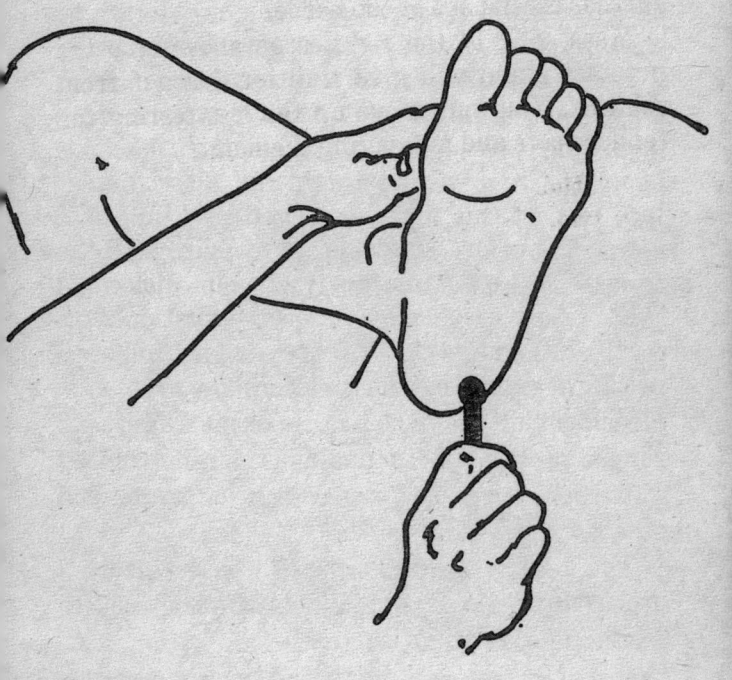

Figure 28.

you must persevere, even if it takes a week or longer.

After you massage the core of the nerve reflex, move up the inner side of the ankle, massaging all the time. This will take care of further extensions of the nerve.

Massaging of the reflexes as shown for the prostate gland will give additional relief from sciatica. You may move up the leg, testing for tender spots and massaging them out.

37

Sore Throat, Loss of Voice

The next time you suffer from a sore throat, try zone therapy instead of sweetened cough pills.

The fleshy part of your big toe is where you will locate the reflex to your throat and, since the pain is in the front part, you will want to massage the top of the toe, just where it merges with your foot. Grab it between your thumb and forefinger and see if it doesn't respond with tenderness the minute you apply some pressure. That should be your tell-tale sign.

The congestion in your throat may be caused by an excessive amount of poison in your system, and if that is the case, that condition will have to be cleared first before you can obtain relief. On the other hand, if you are just catching a cold, you may be surprised at what the proper massage can do for you.

And not only a sore throat but a stiff neck will yield to this approach.

Loss of voice may be helped by using a napkin or handkerchief to grasp the tongue, and pulling it slowly but firmly out and in all directions.

38

Stomach Disorders

One of the worst things that can befall the stomach is the perforation of its internal lining, and the subsequent pain and danger posed by such a condition. Ulcers may be caused by many things; bad food, greasy and hastily eaten, as well as by negative emotional states of being, such as fear and anger. That there is a direct relationship between digestion and the emotions is well known and can be felt by every individual: the butterflies caused by fear and anxiety, the heavy feeling caused by depression, the cramps after undue tension. Something has to be done about the emotions if a cure is going to be effected, but zone therapy can be a powerful aid in bringing back the health of your stomach.

Since the stomach lies fairly high in the abdomen (not far down, as most people think) and somewhat to the left, we can form a pretty good idea of the location of its reflexes in the human foot. Please refer to Figure 11 for the exact area. Begin to explore the area with your thumb or the knuckle of your index finger;

some spots may be more tender than others because the organ is fairly large. Some spots may be really painful, an indication that trouble is brewing. You must then massage that area as softly as you can, increasing the pressure as you see that you can bear the temporary pain. You might be surprised at how quickly stomach troubles react to zone therapy, but you shouldn't be; there are a tremendous number of arteries and veins feeding that area, so that the response to increased circulation can be very vigorous.

Gastric ulcers will respond to firm pressure in the wrists. The front or back of the wrist, if sore, will signify ulcers either in the anterior or the posterior stomach wall. Massage until pain disappears, morning and night. If the ulcer is causing acute pain, try firm pressure on the appropriate fingers for three to fifteen minutes.

The last applies to any abdominal pain, such as that caused by indigestion.

In cases of vomiting, try scratching the thumb and index fingers of the left hand and the first three fingers of the right hand, as well as the webs in between those fingers; also the corresponding sections of the foot.

39

Testes

The reflex to the testes, found below the area marked for the prostate gland in Figure 26, will yield to massage in case of injury or obstruction.

An infection should be treated by reflex massage twice daily until cleared. Dr. FitzGerald emphasizes tongue biting, as it affects all zones and can have an ameliorating effect on any constriction. Rubber bands on all fingers will work just as well.

40

Varicose Veins, Leg Cramps

Zone therapy specialists have found that varicose veins have a connection with the liver and, therefore, they treat the liver reflex in the foot when faced with varicose conditions. The same goes for leg cramps. It is necessary to proceed with some caution at first, since we do not want to activate the liver so much that it releases too many pent-up poisons at one time. Start by massaging the reflex in the right foot for a few seconds morning and night, sensing the degree of tenderness and comparing it to the tenderness the next day. It should decrease slowly, and as it does, the massage can be a little more extensive.

Varicose veins in the rectum have been discussed under the subject of hemorrhoids. All of these are conditions which yield to the proper use of zone therapy.

41

Preventive Therapy—Ten Minutes A Day To Health

Proper and plentiful circulation is the key to health. Your blood just has to get to all parts of the body if it is to remove the many poisons that are secreted by each and every living cell, let alone remove the many dead cells. Modern man does not exercise enough, and when he does, it is through specialized movements that do not take care of every section and muscle of his body. This is the cause of much disease in our time, and it isn't helped by diets too rich in sugars and processed starches and carbohydrates.

There is no substitute for exercise and good dietary habits. But if these rules are observed, and you also take it upon yourself to exercise your glands through zone therapy for just ten minutes a day, we can practically promise you a long, happy life free from the many physical troubles that we see each and every day.

We won't go into the matters of diet and exercise, since such matters would take us too far afield of our purpose in this book. But you have been warned. And let us say that as far as exercise is concerned, many authorities believe the best possible exercise in the world is a good long walk each day. Be sure to carry nothing in your hands. If such a walk can be taken with bare feet on the sandy shore of a sea or a lake, you may be sure that nature itself is doing your zone therapy for you!

But form the habit of rising ten minutes earlier than usual each morning, and of sitting down with your feet up during that time, massaging each and every major reflex we have talked about in this book, with special attention to the areas that are sensitive: those are your future trouble spots.

Begin with your toes and work down to the large pads of the front part of your foot. Don't forget the spine reflex and the various reflexes for the glands, waiting to be brought to maximum performance by this simple expedient. After all, you can exercise your muscles by engaging in a sport, but where is the exercise for for any specific gland? These marvelous structures are supposed to go through life functioning at peak capacity, without the least attention. Unless they go on strike! Then and only then do you start to worry and run to doctors. But why wait, sometimes till it's too late, when a few minutes a day can see you through with buoyant health?

Start the good habit today. If we have done nothing in the writing of this book but convince you of the necessity of exercising your glands through zone therapy then we have succeeded, and your life will take a turn for the better. Good luck, and happy massaging!